Care Without Coverage

Too Little, Too Late

Committee on the Consequences of Uninsurance

Board on Health Care Services

INSTITUTE OF MEDICINE

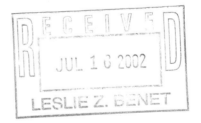
NATIONAL ACADEMY PRESS
Washington, D.C.

NATIONAL ACADEMY PRESS • 2101 Constitution Avenue, N.W. • Washington, DC 20418

NOTICE: The project that is the subject of this report was approved by the Governing Board of the National Research Council, whose members are drawn from the councils of the National Academy of Sciences, the National Academy of Engineering, and the Institute of Medicine. The members of the committee responsible for the report were chosen for their special competences and with regard for appropriate balance.

Support for this project was provided by The Robert Wood Johnson Foundation. The views presented in this report are those of the Institute of Medicine Committee on the Consequences of Uninsurance and are not necessarily those of the funding agencies.

International Standard Book Number 0-309-08343-5

Library of Congress Control Number 2002105905

Additional copies of this report are available for sale from the National Academy Press, 2101 Constitution Avenue, N.W., Box 285, Washington, D.C. 20055. Call (800) 624-6242 or (202) 334-3313 (in the Washington metropolitan area), or visit the NAP's home page at **www.nap.edu.** The full text of this report is available at **www.nap.edu.**

For more information about the Institute of Medicine, visit the IOM home page at **www.iom.edu.**

The serpent has been a symbol of long life, healing, and knowledge among almost all cultures and religions since the beginning of recorded history. The serpent adopted as a logotype by the Institute of Medicine is a relief carving from ancient Greece, now held by the Staatliche Museen in Berlin.

"Knowing is not enough; we must apply.
Willing is not enough; we must do."
—Goethe

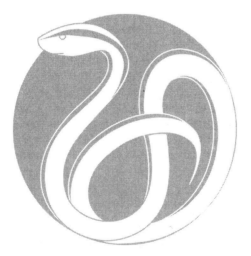

INSTITUTE OF MEDICINE

Shaping the Future for Health

THE NATIONAL ACADEMIES

National Academy of Sciences
National Academy of Engineering
Institute of Medicine
National Research Council

The **National Academy of Sciences** is a private, nonprofit, self-perpetuating society of distinguished scholars engaged in scientific and engineering research, dedicated to the furtherance of science and technology and to their use for the general welfare. Upon the authority of the charter granted to it by the Congress in 1863, the Academy has a mandate that requires it to advise the federal government on scientific and technical matters. Dr. Bruce M. Alberts is president of the National Academy of Sciences.

The **National Academy of Engineering** was established in 1964, under the charter of the National Academy of Sciences, as a parallel organization of outstanding engineers. It is autonomous in its administration and in the selection of its members, sharing with the National Academy of Sciences the responsibility for advising the federal government. The National Academy of Engineering also sponsors engineering programs aimed at meeting national needs, encourages education and research, and recognizes the superior achievements of engineers. Dr. Wm. A. Wulf is president of the National Academy of Engineering.

The **Institute of Medicine** was established in 1970 by the National Academy of Sciences to secure the services of eminent members of appropriate professions in the examination of policy matters pertaining to the health of the public. The Institute acts under the responsibility given to the National Academy of Sciences by its congressional charter to be an adviser to the federal government and, upon its own initiative, to identify issues of medical care, research, and education. Dr. Kenneth I. Shine is president of the Institute of Medicine.

The **National Research Council** was organized by the National Academy of Sciences in 1916 to associate the broad community of science and technology with the Academy's purposes of furthering knowledge and advising the federal government. Functioning in accordance with general policies determined by the Academy, the Council has become the principal operating agency of both the National Academy of Sciences and the National Academy of Engineering in providing services to the government, the public, and the scientific and engineering communities. The Council is administered jointly by both Academies and the Institute of Medicine. Dr. Bruce M. Alberts and Dr. Wm. A. Wulf are chairman and vice chairman, respectively, of the National Research Council.

COMMITTEE ON THE CONSEQUENCES OF UNINSURANCE

IOM Staff

Wilhelmine Miller, Project Co-director
Dianne Miller Wolman, Project Co-director
Lynne Page Snyder, Program Officer
Tracy McKay, Research Associate
Ryan Palugod, Senior Project Assistant

Consultant

Jennifer S. Haas, Assistant Professor of Medicine, San Francisco General
Hospital and University of California, San Francisco

Reviewers

This report has been reviewed in draft form by individuals chosen for their diverse perspectives and technical expertise, in accordance with procedures approved by the NRC's Report Review Committee. The purpose of this independent review is to provide candid and critical comments that will assist the institution in making its published report as sound as possible and to ensure that the report meets institutional standards for objectivity, evidence, and responsiveness to the study charge. The review comments and draft manuscript remain confidential to protect the integrity of the deliberative process. We wish to thank the following individuals for their review of this report:

GERARD ANDERSON, Director, Center for Hospital Finance and Management, Johns Hopkins Health System, Baltimore, MD

JEREMIAH A. BARONDESS, President, New York Academy of Medicine, New York

ANDREW BINDMAN, Associate Professor, Epidemiology and Biostatistics, University of California, San Francisco

DANA GOLDMAN, Senior Economist, RAND Health Communications, Director, UCLA/RAND Health Services Research Postdoctoral Training Program, Santa Monica

NICOLE LURIE, Senior Natural Scientist and Paul O'Neill Alcoa Professor, RAND Corporation, Arlington, VA

DIANE MAKUC, Director, Division of Health and Utilization Analysis, National Center for Health Statistics, Hyattsville, MD

DAVID MECHANIC, Director, Institute for Health, Health Care Policy, and Aging Research, Rutgers, The State University of New Jersey – New Brunswick

THOMAS SCHELLING, Distinguished University Professor, School of Public Affairs, University of Maryland, College Park

RICHARD SORIAN, Director of Public Affairs and Senior Researcher, Center for Studying Health System Change, Washington, DC

DAVID R. WILLIAMS, Professor of Sociology and Senior Research Scientist, Survey Research Center, Institute for Social Research, University of Michigan, Ann Arbor

Although the reviewers listed above have provided many constructive comments and suggestions, they were not asked to endorse the conclusions or recommendations nor did they see the final draft of the report before its release. The review of this report was overseen by **Hugh H. Tilson, Clinical Professor, School of Public Health, University of North Carolina, Chapel Hill,** appointed by the Institute of Medicine and **Charles E. Phelps, Provost, University of Rochester,** appointed by the NRC's Report Review Committee, who were responsible for making certain that an independent examination of this report was carried out in accordance with institutional procedures and that all review comments were carefully considered. Responsibility for the final content of this report rests entirely with the authoring committee and the institution.

Foreword

Care Without Coverage: Too Little, Too Late appears at a critical juncture in our national health policy debate. It comes when, for the first time, legislators and other policy makers are not disputing the need to help individuals and families maintain health insurance coverage during economic downturns, but only the best strategies for doing so. This second report of the Institute of Medicine (IOM) Committee on the Consequences of Uninsurance confirms what most health care professionals have long believed and the general American public has acted upon: *health insurance makes a difference in people's lives.* The public has acted upon this premise by taking up workplace health insurance, buying individual policies, and enrolling in publicly sponsored plans when they qualify for them. This practical evidence of the value Americans place on having health insurance coexists, paradoxically, with the commonly held belief (discussed in depth in the Committee's first report, *Coverage Matters: Insurance and Health Care*, and briefly in this report) that Americans without health insurance manage to get the care that they really need.

Care Without Coverage should disabuse all of us of this overly optimistic view of how health care operates for the 40 million uninsured Americans. It provides a critical and comprehensive review of research on the effects of health insurance coverage or its lack for adults in the United States. The authoring Committee and its Subcommittee on Health Outcomes for the Uninsured have produced a report that responds with well-documented evidence to the assumption and assertion that health insurance is not an essential component of access to quality health care or to healthy outcomes in America. In this country, we do not see many people dying in the streets because of inaccessible health care, and it has been easy to assume that people without health insurance manage to get the care they need.

The report refutes this assumption by delineating in some detail how the health of adults who do not have health insurance is compromised by their lack of coverage. This report constitutes important new information for national and state policy makers as they deliberate about health, economic, and social welfare policy. What is at stake is not only the health of those without health insurance but our nation's reputation and character as a fair and compassionate society.

The Institute of Medicine is grateful to The Robert Wood Johnson Foundation for supporting this series of reports addressing the personal and social impacts of uninsurance.

Kenneth I. Shine, M.D.
President, Institute of Medicine
May 2002

Preface

This is the second report in a series of six that the Institute of Medicine (IOM) Committee on the Consequences of Uninsurance is issuing. The Committee's first report, *Coverage Matters: Insurance and Health Care,* was released in October 2001. It provides an overview of health insurance in the United States, describes the dynamic and often unstable nature of coverage, identifies the characteristics of Americans who are likely to lack health insurance, and delineates the scope of the problem of uninsurance in this country. *Coverage Matters* is a timely contribution to the ongoing policy debates about health insurance, and we commend our initial report to your attention along with this current one.

Care Without Coverage: Too Little, Too Late builds on the foundation of information and analysis laid in the first report and examines the question of the health consequences for adults who lack health insurance. *Care Without Coverage* is based on a focused and critical review of clinical and epidemiological research that sheds light on the question of whether and how having health insurance or lacking it affects the care adults receive and their health status as a result. The Committee's work led it to the conclusion that health insurance does, indeed, make a significant difference in the health of American adults and that uninsured adults experience worse health as a consequence of their lack of coverage.

The research, analysis, and preparation of *Care Without Coverage* involved the committed efforts of Committee members, IOM staff, and consultants to the project. The Subcommittee on Health Outcomes for the Uninsured, chaired by Edward Wagner, designed and conducted the critical review of research studies upon which the Committee based its findings and conclusions. Committee members Ronald Andersen, John Ayanian, and Edward Wagner were joined on the subcommittee by Paula Diehr, David Meltzer, Cynthia Mulrow, and Robin

Weinick, members who enhanced and deepened the expertise available to the Committee in its work on this study. We are deeply indebted to the intensive efforts of the Subcommittee in the analysis and drafting of this report. IOM staff members Wilhelmine Miller, the principal analyst on this report, Tracy McKay, Lynne Snyder, Dianne Wolman and Ryan Palugod supported the Committee and Subcommittee in all aspects of their work, and this report reflects their dedication and initiative. As primary consultant to the Committee, Jennifer Haas helped to clarify the complex issues of the overlapping influence of race and ethnicity, socioeconomic status, and health insurance on health outcomes, and we are grateful for her generous participation in the Committee's work.

We hope that *Care Without Coverage: Too Little, Too Late* will contribute to the current public examination of options for the stabilization and expansion of health insurance coverage and improvements in access to care for all of our nation's people. The Committee's next report, which examines impacts of uninsurance on the family and health outcomes for children, pregnant women, and newborns, will be released this fall. The final three Committee reports—on community impacts of uninsured populations, societal economic costs, and models and criteria for health financing reforms—will be released in the winter, spring, and fall of 2003, respectively. Each of these reports will provide policy makers and the American public with solid new information and insights to inform decision making about health insurance coverage at every level.

Finally, we would like to thank The Robert Wood Johnson Foundation for its continued support of the Committee's work.

> Mary Sue Coleman, Ph.D.
> *Co-chair*
> Arthur Kellermann, M.D., M.P.H.
> *Co-chair*
> May 2002

Acknowledgments

Care Without Coverage: Too Little, Too Late benefited from the contributions of many people. The Committee takes this opportunity to recognize those who helped it develop the analyses on which the report is based.

The Committee particularly acknowledges the members of the Subcommittee on Health Outcomes for the Uninsured, which developed this report: Edward Wagner (chair), Ronald Andersen, John Ayanian, Paula Diehr, David Meltzer, Cynthia Mulrow, and Robin Weinick. All members of the Subcommittee contributed much time and advice in designing the critical literature review that supports this report's findings and conclusions, and in reviewing and critiquing scores of primary research articles themselves.

Jennifer Haas served as a principal consultant to the Subcommittee and, with Nancy Adler, professor of medical psychology at the University of California at San Fransisco (UCSF) and chair of the MacArthur Research Network on Socioeconomic Status and Health, prepared a background paper that analyzed how race, ethnicity, and socioeconomic factors contribute to differences in health outcomes and how these factors should be taken into account in interpreting findings about health insurance effects. Jennifer generously gave her time for conference calls and meetings during the preparation of this report, and her expertise informs it throughout.

Michael Feuerstein, professor of medical and clinical psychology, preventive medicine and biometrics at the Uniformed Services University of the Health Sciences, Bethesda, Maryland, contributed his time and expertise to the Committee by analyzing and synthesizing the research on mental health care and outcomes and health insurance. Linda Kohn and Elaine Swift, senior program officers in the Division of Health Care Services, Institute of Medicine, also participated in the primary literature review and evaluation effort, and advised project staff on its interpretation. Consulting editor Cheryl Ulmer assisted in preparation of the Executive Summary.

Highly expert and accomplished consultants were enlisted in the effort to critically review more than 130 research studies within a six-week time frame last summer. Consultants to the Committee who served in this capacity were Margot Kushel, assistant professor of medicine, UCSF; Marcia Polansky, associate professor of biostatistics, Drexel University; Joshua Sarver, Center for Health Care Research and Policy, Case Western Reserve University; and Dean Schillinger, associate professor of medicine, UCSF. The Committee is very grateful for their thoughtful and thorough critiques and their willingness to contribute to this project.

The Committee recognizes the hard work of staff at the Institute of Medicine. This work is conducted under the guidance of Janet Corrigan, director, Board on Health Care Services. All members of the project team, directed by Wilhelmine Miller and Dianne Wolman, contributed to this report. Wilhelmine was lead staff in working with the Subcommittee and Committee in developing and managing the critical literature review and in drafting *Care Without Coverage*. Dianne and Program Officer Lynne Snyder reviewed and edited multiple drafts and background documents and contributed in many ways to the final report. In addition to summarizing studies and collecting the large number of articles and references acquired for this report, Research Associate Tracy McKay resourcefully conducted numerous systematic literature searches under the Subcommittee's direction and identified many published studies that might otherwise have been missed. She also prepared the manuscript for publication. Senior Project Assistant Ryan Palugod efficiently supported communications with Committee members, handled meeting logistics, and managed the numerous consultancy arrangements related to the literature review.

Funding for the project comes from The Robert Wood Johnson Foundation (RWJF). The committee extends special thanks to Steven Schroeder, president, and Anne Weiss, senior program officer, RWJF, for their continuing support and interest in this project.

Finally, the Committee would like to thank co-chairs Mary Sue Coleman and Arthur Kellermann for their guidance and Subcommittee Chair Edward Wagner for his leadership in the research and development of *Care Without Coverage*.

Contents

APPENDIXES

Care Without Coverage

Too Little, Too Late

BOX ES-1
Review of Committee Findings

This is a brief overview of the Committee's specific findings regarding the effects of insurance on the health of American adults. The Committee's overall conclusions are presented at the end of the Executive Summary.

Prevention and Screening

• Uninsured adults are less likely than adults with any kind of health coverage to receive preventive and screening services and to receive them on a timely basis. Health insurance that provides coverage of preventive and screening services is likely to result in greater and more appropriate use of these services.
• Health insurance would likely reduce racial and ethnic disparities in the receipt of preventive and screening services.

Cancer

• Uninsured cancer patients generally are in poorer health and are more likely to die prematurely than persons with insurance, largely because of delayed diagnosis. This finding is supported by population-based studies of persons with breast, cervical, colorectal, and prostate cancer and melanoma.

Chronic Illness

• Uninsured adults living with chronic diseases are less likely to receive appropriate care to manage their health conditions than are those who have health insurance. For the five disease conditions that the Committee examined (diabetes, cardiovascular disease, end-stage renal disease, HIV infection, and mental illness), uninsured patients have consistently worse clinical outcomes than insured patients.
• Uninsured adults with diabetes are less likely to receive recommended services. Lacking health insurance for longer periods increases the risk of inadequate care for this condition and can lead to uncontrolled blood sugar levels, which, over time, put diabetics at risk for additional chronic disease and disability.
• Uninsured adults with hypertension or high blood cholesterol have diminished access to care, are less likely to be screened, are less likely to take prescription medication if diagnosed, and experience worse health outcomes.
• Uninsured patients with end-stage renal disease begin dialysis with more severe disease than do those who had insurance before beginning dialysis.
• Uninsured adults with HIV infection are less likely to receive highly effective medications that have been shown to improve survival and die sooner than those with coverage.
• Adults with health insurance that covers any mental health treatment are more likely to receive mental health services and care consistent with clinical practice guidelines than are those without any health insurance or with insurance that does not cover mental health conditions.

Hospital-Based Care

• Uninsured patients who are hospitalized for a range of conditions are more likely to die in the hospital, to receive fewer services when admitted, and to experience substandard care and resultant injury than are insured patients.

• Uninsured persons with trauma are less likely to be admitted to the hospital, more likely to receive fewer services when admitted, and are more likely to die than are insured trauma victims.

• Uninsured patients with acute cardiovascular disease are less likely to be admitted to a hospital that performs angiography or revascularization procedures, are less likely to receive these diagnostic and treatment procedures, and are more likely to die in the short term. Health insurance reduces the disparity in receipt of these services by members of racial and ethnic minority groups.

General Health Status

• Relatively short (one- to four-year) longitudinal studies document relatively greater decreases in general health status measures for uninsured adults and for those who lost insurance coverage during the period studied than for those with continuous coverage.

• Longitudinal population-based studies of the mortality of uninsured and privately insured adults reveal a higher risk of dying prematurely for those who were uninsured at the beginning of the study than for those who initially had private coverage.

Executive Summary

This report, the second in a series of six planned by the Institute of Medicine (IOM) Committee on the Consequences of Uninsurance, examines the relationship between being insured or uninsured and the health of American adults. *Care Without Coverage: Too Little, Too Late* follows the issuance last October of *Coverage Matters: Insurance and Health Care*, which provided an overview of health insurance in the United States, described the dynamic and frequently unstable nature of coverage, and delineated the extent of uninsurance and the characteristics of Americans who are most likely to be uninsured. Over the next 15 months the Committee will issue reports on family, community, and economic impacts of uninsurance and, last, a report that identifies models and strategies for addressing the problem of uninsurance.

Contrary to popular belief, Americans who do not have health insurance are at risk for poorer health as a result of their lack of coverage. In its first report, *Coverage Matters: Insurance and Health Care*, the Committee presented several popular myths about the lack of health insurance that indicated considerable public misunderstanding about the importance of coverage, which has hampered efforts to advance solutions. In 1999 almost 60 percent of the public believed that uninsured people get the health care they need from doctors and hospitals. The reality is that those without health insurance are much more likely to go without care than are people who have insurance (IOM, 2001a). In this report, the Committee examines whether this reduced access to care results in less appropriate care and poor health consequences.

Ascertaining whether health insurance improves health outcomes is critical to shaping public policy about health insurance and the financing of health care more generally. The strongest research studies consistently show that working-age Americans (those between 18 and 65) who do not have health insurance have poorer health and die prematurely. The Committee concludes that if these roughly 30 million working-age Americans were to become insured on a continuous basis, their health would be expected to improve.

Increasingly, clinical and health services research provides evidence that receiving too little medical care or receiving it too late has harmful effects for those without health insurance. These effects could be ameliorated through the enhanced access to care that insurance provides. In this report the Committee weighs the evidence of the effect of being uninsured on health-related outcomes for adults and considers the potential benefits of extending health insurance to adults without it. In a subsequent report, the Committee will examine comparable studies focused on children.

Being uninsured is associated with a variety of worse health-related outcomes, including the following:

- less frequent or no use of cancer screening tests resulting in delayed diagnosis and premature mortality for cancer patients (Ayanian et al., 1993; Roetzheim et al., 1999, 2000a, 2000b; Ferrante et al., 2000; Breen et al., 2001; Perkins et al., 2001);
- care that does not meet professionally recommended standards for the management of chronic disease, for example, the failure of persons with diabetes to receive timely eye and foot exams to prevent blindness and amputations (Beckles et al., 1998; Ayanian et al., 2000);
- lack of access to and maintenance of appropriate medication regimens for persons with hypertension or HIV infection (W.E. Cunningham et al., 1995, 1999, 2000; Shapiro et al., 1999; Huttin et al., 2000; Goldman et al., 2001); and
- fewer diagnostic and treatment services for trauma or heart attacks and an increased risk of death when in the hospital (Haas and Goldman, 1994; Blustein et al., 1995; Canto et al., 1999, 2000; Doyle, 2001).

The health benefits of having insurance are even stronger when continuity of coverage is taken into account. Being uninsured for relatively short periods (one to four years) appears to result in a decrease in general health status. When followed over longer periods of time, uninsured adults have been found to be at higher risk of premature death than are persons with private coverage (Lurie et al., 1984, 1986; Franks et al., 1993a; Sorlie et al., 1994; Baker et al., 2001).

Additionally, the potential health benefits of having insurance are magnified when vulnerable populations, already at increased risk of worse health, receive coverage. These vulnerable groups include adults who are

- chronically ill (especially between the ages of 55 and 64 years),
- living with severe mental illness,
- members of racial and ethnic minority groups, and
- of lower socioeconomic status.

Based on the preponderance of evidence, the Committee concludes that

- the health of uninsured adults is worse than it would otherwise be if they were insured,
- providing health insurance to uninsured adults would result in improved health, including greater life expectancy, and
- increased rates of health insurance coverage would especially improve the health of those in the poorest health and most disadvantaged in terms of access to care and thus would likely reduce health disparities among racial and ethnic groups.

ASSESSING THE IMPACT OF HEALTH INSURANCE ON HEALTH

The Committee reached these conclusions after a review that used explicit criteria to select and evaluate the best-designed research studies investigating the health of working-age adults with and without health insurance. To be selected, studies had to consider (1) an individual's health insurance status as an independent variable or "predictor," and (2) the effect of insurance status on one or more health-related outcomes for adults ages 18 through 64. A subsequent report will review the effects of health insurance coverage on children and on pregnant women. Studies that focus primarily on adults 65 years and older were excluded because virtually all in this age group have health insurance coverage through the federal Medicare program.[1]

This report uses specific definitions of insurance and of the terms of coverage. "Insured adults" means those with general medical and hospitalization insurance, while "uninsured adults" are persons without *any* health insurance. The Committee has not explicitly considered those who may be inadequately insured ("underinsured"). Although the Committee did not examine studies comparing benefit packages among those with insurance or set out to analyze distinctions among kinds of health insurance, the literature led it to consider some features of health insurance that appear to affect health outcomes. For example, distinctive results from studies that compared those with private and public health insurance point to characteristics such as continuity of coverage and coverage of prescription drugs as important factors. The Committee paid particular attention to studies that examined the length of time participants were uninsured to determine whether and how that factor affected health.

---

[1] While Medicare covers hospitalizations, physician, and other outpatient services including rehabilitative therapies and home health care, it does not cover most outpatient prescription drugs nor does it cover nonrehabilitative long-term care.

Because most of the evidence comes from studies that are observational rather than experimental, interpreting the evidence about the value of coverage for health outcomes requires application of careful standards of analysis and review. Consequently, analytical adjustments are required to account for potential biases related to variation among study subjects in lengths of time uninsured, types of health insurance coverage, and characteristics of study participants that correlate with health insurance status whose effects can be confused or confounded with those of insurance.

Three characteristics of individuals are closely related to health insurance status and, as a result, require analytic adjustment: health status, race and ethnicity, and socioeconomic status. The strongest observational studies use adjustments to separate the effects of these characteristics from those of health insurance coverage.

The Committee believes that the research literature likely understates the differences in health outcomes between insured and uninsured adults that can be attributed to health insurance. One of the shortcomings in the literature is a lack of information about the experience of those adults who do not seek care, whether insured or uninsured. Research that relies on administrative or clinical documentation of health care use cannot account for the experience of those who do not seek treatment, and uninsured adults are less likely to seek treatment than are insured adults. Thus, studies that rely on health care records to compare groups may actually overstate the utilization of services by uninsured populations.

> **Finding: Health insurance coverage is associated with better health outcomes for adults. It is also associated with having a regular source of care and with greater and more appropriate use of health services. These factors, in turn, improve the likelihood of disease screening and early detection, the management of chronic illness, and the effective treatment of acute conditions such as traumatic injury and heart attacks. The ultimate result is improved health outcomes.**

Health insurance makes a difference in receipt of services and health outcomes. Direct measures of health examined in studies include self-reported health status, mortality, stage of disease at time of diagnosis, and physiologic measures (e.g., controlled blood pressure in persons with hypertension). Because direct measures of health outcomes are often hard to obtain inexpensively in large-scale studies, intermediate measures of health care processes are commonly used as proxies to assess the effect of health insurance on health. This report examines receipt of recommended services, for example, dilated eye exams annually for persons with diabetes and regular blood pressure checks for those with hypertension, that have been validated by professional guidelines and clinical effectiveness research.

Finding: Health insurance is most likely to improve health outcomes if it is continuous and links people to appropriate health care. When health insurance includes preventive and screening services, prescription drugs, and mental health care, it is more strongly associated with the receipt of appropriate care than when insurance does not have these features.

Adults without health insurance face serious shortcomings in access to care. The quality and length of life are distinctly different for insured and uninsured populations, with worse health status and shortened lives among uninsured adults. While having health insurance demonstrably increases use of services, more importantly, it also facilitates more appropriate use of health care services. In prevention and chronic disease management for example, having health insurance greatly increases the likelihood of a regular source of care and of continuity in care, which in turn can improve health outcomes.

Finding: Increased health insurance coverage would likely reduce racial and ethnic disparities in the use of appropriate health care services and may also reduce disparities in morbidity and mortality among ethnic groups.

Members of different racial and ethnic groups differ in terms of health status, the likelihood of having health insurance, and the care that they receive (Haas and Adler, 2001; IOM, 2001a, 2002; Mills, 2001). Health insurance does not eliminate all disparities among population groups in access to care or remediate all deficits in health status among minority populations. It does, however, facilitate receipt of preventive services, having a regular source of care, and improved quality of care.

EFFECTS OF HEALTH INSURANCE ON SPECIFIC HEALTH CONDITIONS

In the following discussion of health services and conditions, the evidence reviewed by the Committee is presented as follows:

- primary prevention and screening services;
- cancer care and outcomes;
- chronic disease care and outcomes (including diabetes, cardiovascular disease, end-stage renal disease, HIV infection, and mental illness);
- hospital-based care (including trauma care and care for coronary artery disease);
- general health outcomes.

Primary Prevention and Screening Services

Finding: Uninsured adults are less likely than adults with any kind of health coverage to receive preventive and screening services and to receive these services on a timely basis. Health insurance that provides more extensive coverage of preventive and screening services is likely to result in greater and more appropriate use of these services.

Uninsured adults are less likely than those with health insurance to receive preventive services such as mammograms, clinical breast exams, Pap tests, and colorectal screening (Powell-Griner et al., 1999; Ayanian et al., 2000, Breen et al., 2001). The positive effect of having insurance is more evident with relatively costly services such as mammograms (Zambrana et al., 1999; Cummings et al., 2000). Studies of particular ethnic groups find that health insurance is associated with the increased receipt of preventive services and an increased likelihood of having a regular source of care (Mandelblatt et al., 1999).

Generally, insurance benefits are less likely to include preventive and screening services than physician visits for acute care or diagnostic tests for symptomatic conditions. The more extensive the coverage of preventive services, the more likely are health plan enrollees to receive these services (Faulkner and Schauffler, 1997). Yet even if people have health insurance that does not cover preventive services, they are more likely to receive appropriate services than are those without any form of health insurance, partly because they are more likely to have a regular source of care or a primary provider.

Even after adjustments for age, race, education, and regular source of care, uninsured adults are less likely to receive timely screening for breast, cervical, or colorectal cancer. Once discovered, their cancer is likely to be at a more advanced stage.

Cancer Care and Outcomes

Finding: Uninsured cancer patients die sooner, on average, than do persons with insurance, largely because of delayed diagnosis. This finding is supported by population-based studies of breast, cervical, colorectal, and prostate cancer and melanoma.

Uninsured cancer patients more often fare poorly than do patients with coverage. A relatively advanced, often fatal, late stage of disease at the time of diagnosis is more common among persons without insurance coverage, reflecting their reduced use of timely screening services. Uninsured persons with breast, colorectal, or prostate cancer are more likely to die prematurely from their disease than are patients with private health insurance. For example, uninsured women with breast cancer have a risk of dying that is between 30 and 50 percent higher than the risk for women with private health insurance (Ayanian et al., 1993; Lee-Feldstein et al., 2000; Roetzheim et al., 2000a), and uninsured patients with colorectal cancer are about 50 percent more likely to die than are patients with private coverage, even when the cancer is diagnosed at similar stages (Roetzheim et al., 2000b). This evidence comes from research using area or statewide cancer registries.

Uninsured adults with cancer might experience differences in treatment. For example, uninsured women with breast cancer are less likely than privately insured women to receive breast-conserving surgery (Roetzheim et al., 2000a). It should be noted, however, that disparities in treatment persist among racial and ethnic groups even if all have insurance (IOM, 2002).

Chronic Disease Care and Outcomes

Finding: Uninsured adults living with chronic diseases are less likely to receive appropriate care to manage their health conditions than are those who have health insurance. For all five disease conditions (in addition to cancer) that the Committee examined (diabetes, cardiovascular disease, end-stage renal disease, HIV infection and mental illness), uninsured patients have consistently worse clinical outcomes than do insured patients.

For persons living with a chronic illness, health insurance may be most important in enhancing opportunities to acquire a regular source of care and receive appropriate management of their condition. Identifying chronic conditions early and providing professionally recommended, cost-effective interventions on an ongoing and coordinated basis can improve health outcomes. Yet uninsured adults with chronic conditions are less likely to have a usual source of care or regular check-ups than are chronically ill persons with coverage (Ayanian et al., 2000; Fish-Parcham, 2001).

Diabetes

Uninsured persons with diabetes are less likely to receive recommended services. Lacking health insurance for longer periods increases the risk of inadequate care for this condition and can lead to uncontrolled blood sugar levels, which, over time, put diabetics at risk for additional chronic disease and disability. Despite the demanding and costly care regimen that persons with diabetes face, adults with diabetes are almost as likely to be uninsured as adults without this disease (12 percent are uninsured compared to the general population uninsured rate of 15 percent [Harris, 1999].)

Uninsured adults with diabetes are less likely to receive the recommended professional standard of care than those with health insurance. For example, they are less likely to receive regular foot or dilated eye exams that are important in the prevention of foot ulcers and blindness. Twenty-five percent of adults with diabetes who were uninsured for a year or more went without a checkup within the past two years, compared to 7 percent of diabetics who were uninsured for less than a year and 5 percent of diabetics with health insurance (Beckles et al., 1998; Ayanian et al., 2000).

Cardiovascular Disease

Uninsured adults with hypertension or high cholesterol have diminished access to care, are less likely to be screened, are less likely to take prescription medication if diagnosed, and experience worse health.

According to analyses of national health survey data, 19 percent of uninsured adults with heart disease and 13 percent with hypertension lack a usual source of care, compared to 8 and 4 percent, respectively, of their insured counterparts (Fish-Parcham, 2001). Uninsured adults have less frequent monitoring of blood pressure once they are diagnosed with hypertension and are less likely to stay on drug therapy than are insured adults who have hypertension (Huttin et al., 2000; Fish-Parcham, 2001).

Loss of insurance coverage disrupts therapeutic relationships and worsens blood pressure control (Lurie et al., 1984, 1986). Deficits in care for uninsured adults with hypertension or high cholesterol place them at risk of complications and deterioration of their condition. For example, patients admitted to emergency departments with severe uncontrolled hypertension were more likely to be uninsured than socio-demographically similar patients with any insurance (Shea et al., 1992a, 1992b).

End-Stage Renal Disease

Uninsured patients have more severe renal failure when they begin dialysis than insured patients (Kausz et al., 2000). The clinical goals for patients with kidney disease are to slow the progression of renal failure, manage complications, and prevent or manage coexisting disease effectively. Uninsured patients are less likely than insured patients to have received treatment for related anemia before initiating dialysis, and their health status is already compromised by a greater likelihood of more severe anemia (Obrador et al., 1999).

The virtually universal qualification of end-stage renal disease (ESRD) patients for Medicare once dialysis or transplantation becomes necessary erases previously existing gender and racial or ethnic disparities in access to hospital-based care for ESRD patients with heart disease (Daumit et al., 1999, 2000).

Human Immunodeficiency Virus Infection

Uninsured adults, once diagnosed with HIV, face greater delays in accessing appropriate care than those with health insurance and are more likely to forgo needed care. Persons without health insurance have been shown to wait more than three months after diagnosis to have their first office visit and to wait an average of four months longer than privately insured patients to receive newer drug therapies (Turner et al., 2000). Furthermore, the uninsured with HIV are less likely to be able to maintain a recommended drug regimen over time (Cunningham et al., 2000).

Uninsured adults with HIV infection are less likely to receive highly effective medications that have become the standard of treatment within the past five years and been shown to improve survival (Carpenter et al., 1996, 1998; Goldman et al., 2001). Having health insurance of any kind has been found to reduce mortality in HIV-infected adults by 71–85 percent over a six-month period, with the greater reduction found more recently when effective drug therapies were in more widespread use (Goldman et al., 2001).

Mental Illness

Adults with health insurance that covers any mental health treatment are more likely to receive mental health services and care consistent with clinical practice guidelines than are those without any health insurance or with insurance that does not cover mental health conditions.

Mental illness represents a major but often underestimated source of disability and is equivalent to heart disease and cancer in terms of its impact. Depression and anxiety disorders are often treatable in the general medical sector and primarily require outpatient services. Severe mental illnesses (schizophrenia, other psychoses, and bipolar depression) require the attention of specialty mental health professionals and may require more extensive services (e.g., inpatient services, partial or day hospitalization).

Receipt of appropriate care has been associated with improved functional outcomes for depression and anxiety disorders, yet the uninsured are less likely to receive this degree of care. Patients without health insurance for mental health visits who were diagnosed with depression, panic disorder, or generalized anxiety disorder were less likely to receive mental health services (Druss and Rosenheck, 1998; Cooper-Patrick et al., 1999). When they did receive care, it was less likely to be appropriate (concordant with professional practice guidelines) (Wang et al., 2000; Young et al., 2001). Uninsured adults with severe mental illnesses also receive less appropriate care or medications and experience delays in receiving services until they gain public insurance coverage (Rabinowitz et al., 1998, 2001; McAlpine and Mechanic, 2000).

Even when health insurance does not specifically cover mental health services, having it increases the likelihood that someone with depression or anxiety will receive some care for the condition. Persons with a severe mental illness such as schizophrenia or bipolar disorder face difficulties in obtaining and then keeping health insurance after diagnosis. When they do have health insurance, especially public insurance (Medicare or Medicaid), they are more likely to receive specialty mental health services than are severely ill persons without any health insurance or even patients with private insurance.

Hospital-Based Care

Finding: Uninsured patients who are hospitalized for a range of conditions are more likely to die in the hospital, to receive fewer services, and, when admitted, are more likely to experience substandard care and resultant injury than are insured patients.

Poorer health status for uninsured adults when they are hospitalized is compounded by their experiences as inpatients. Being uninsured is associated with the receipt of fewer needed services, worse quality care, and greater risk of dying in the hospital or shortly after discharge (Hadley et al., 1991; Burstin et al., 1992; Haas and Goldman, 1994; Blustein et al., 1995; Doyle, 2001). Being uninsured and not having a regular source of care are also associated with delays in seeking care from the emergency department for a variety of conditions, delays that may compromise outcomes (e.g., rupture in acute appendicitis) (Braveman et al., 1994).

Because most hospital-based studies are biased by the inclusion of self-selected patients who "show up" for care, the Committee decided to focus on two conditions—traumatic injuries and acute cardiac events—for which most people receive hospital care whether or not they are insured.

Traumatic Injuries

Uninsured persons with traumatic injuries are less likely to be admitted to the hospital, receive fewer services when admitted, and are more likely to die than are insured trauma victims.

Provider response to traumatic injury can be influenced by insurance status. In one statewide study of uninsured auto accident victims, uninsured patients were found to receive less care and had a 37 percent higher mortality rate than did privately insured accident victims (Doyle, 2001). Another statewide study showed while uninsured trauma patients were as likely to receive intensive care unit services as privately insured patients, they were less likely to undergo operative procedures or receive physical therapy (Haas and Goldman, 1994).

Acute Cardiovascular Disease

Uninsured patients with acute cardiovascular disease are less likely to be admitted to a hospital that performs angiography or revascularization procedures, are less likely to receive these diagnostic and treatment procedures, and are more likely to die in the short term. Health insurance reduces the disparity in receipt of these services for women relative to men and for members of racial and ethnic minority groups (Carlisle et al., 1997; Daumit et al., 1999, 2000).

Insurance status influences the receipt of hospital-based treatments for cardiovascular disease (specifically, coronary artery disease). Uninsured patients hospitalized for acute myocardial infarction (heart attack) experience a greater risk of dying during their hospital stay or shortly thereafter than do patients with private insurance (Young and Cohen, 1991; Blustein et al., 1995; Canto et al., 2000).

The choice of hospital itself has significant effects on diagnosis, treatment, and health-related outcomes. Uninsured patients are less likely to be admitted to a hospital that performs angiography or cardiac revascularization (Leape et al., 1999) and are less likely to receive these diagnostic and treatment procedures regardless of hospital facilities (Canto et al., 1999). Insurance status has also been shown to influence access to transfers for revascularization (Blustein et al., 1995).

GENERAL HEALTH OUTCOMES

An uninsured adult's experiences with ambulatory and hospital care influence his or her health status in important ways over the short term and may lead to a premature death.

Health Status

Finding: Relatively short (one- to four-year) longitudinal studies document decreases in general health status measures for uninsured adults and for those who lost insurance coverage compared to persons with continuous coverage.

Like those with chronic health conditions, adults in late middle age are more likely to experience declines in function and health status if they lack or lose health insurance coverage (Baker et al., 2001). Changes in health status might include worsening control of blood pressure, decreased ability to walk or climb stairs, or decline of general self-perceived wellness and functioning. The effect of being uninsured on self-reported health measures is greater for lower-income persons (Franks et al., 1993b).

Mortality

Finding: Longitudinal population-based studies of the mortality of uninsured and privately insured adults reveal a higher risk of dying for those who were uninsured at the beginning of the study than for those who initially had private coverage.

Longer-term population-based studies (from 5 to 17 years) find a 25 percent higher risk of dying for adults who were uninsured at the beginning of the study (Franks et al., 1993a; Sorlie et al., 1994). These analyses of overall mortality are corroborated by the mortality experience of insured and uninsured patients with heart attack, cancer, traumatic injury, and HIV infection (Blustein et al., 1995; Canto et al., 2000; Ayanian et al., 1993; Roetzheim et al., 2000a; Doyle, 2001; Goldman et al., 2001).

THE DIFFERENCE COVERAGE COULD MAKE TO THE HEALTH OF UNINSURED ADULTS

Particular groups of uninsured adults are more likely to experience poor health or barriers to care and thus can be expected to benefit more from gaining health insurance. These groups include uninsured adults who are chronically ill, persons with severe mental illness, members of some racial and ethnic minority groups, and persons with lower socioeconomic status. Many of the uninsured belong to one or more of these higher-risk groups.

The Committee bases the following summary conclusions on the substantial consistency of results among the methodologically strongest observational studies in its review and the coherence of these results with the behavioral research that informs the Committee's conceptual model of mechanisms by which health insurance affects health outcomes:

• **Having health insurance is associated with better health outcomes for adults and with their receipt of appropriate care across a range of preventive, chronic, and acute care services. Adults without health insurance coverage die sooner and experience greater declines in health status over time than do adults with continuous coverage.**

• **Adults with chronic conditions and those in late middle age stand to benefit the most from health insurance coverage in terms of improved health outcomes because of their high probability of needing health care services.**

• **Population groups that most often lack stable health insurance coverage and that have worse health status, including racial and ethnic minorities and lower-income adults, would benefit most from increased health insurance coverage. Increased coverage would likely reduce some of the racial and ethnic disparities in the utilization of appropriate health care services and may also reduce disparities in morbidity and mortality among ethnic groups.**

• **Health insurance that affords access to providers and includes preventive and screening services, outpatient prescription drugs, and specialty mental health care is more likely to facilitate the receipt of appropriate care.**

• **Broad-based health insurance strategies across the entire uninsured population would be more likely to produce these benefits than would "rescue" programs aimed only at the seriously ill.**

What differences in health care utilization and outcomes would health insurance make if the uninsured were provided with coverage? Despite the scarcity of experiments testing the impacts of providing health insurance to the previously uninsured, the Committee believes that the powerful and consistent observational evidence across a wide variety of populations and health conditions, corroborated by the few experimental and quasi-experimental studies that have been conducted, provides a reasonable basis for answering this question.

The key lies in the role health insurance can play in facilitating access to care and the timely and appropriate use of services. In addition, if uninsured adults were insured on a continuous basis, their health status would likely be better than it would be otherwise and their risk of dying prematurely would be reduced. The survival benefits derived from insurance coverage, however, can be achieved in full only when health insurance is acquired well before the development of advanced disease. The problem of later diagnosis and higher mortality among uninsured women with breast cancer, for example, cannot be solved by insuring women once their disease is diagnosed (Perkins et al., 2001).

Finally, the evidence presented accounts only for some of the benefits and advantages that health insurance provides. Financial risk reduction and economic security are major benefits that accrue to everyone with coverage, whether or not they use it (IOM, 2001a). Patient satisfaction and the sense of being valued when professional and caring attention is provided in painful, stressful, or frightening circumstances are genuine, desirable outcomes. These qualities are more likely to be found in health care settings and healing relationships where one is confident of good access to health care providers' time and resources. Adults without health insurance are less likely to feel deserving of a physician's attention when they seek care, and indeed, uninsured adults are less likely to seek needed care than are those with health insurance. Financial security and stability, peace of mind, alleviation of pain and suffering, improved physical function, disabilities avoided or delayed, and gains in life expectancy constitute an array of health insurance benefits that accrue to members of our society who have health insurance. For many of the 40 million uninsured Americans, these benefits remain out of reach.

1

Introduction

What are the health consequences for the roughly 30 million (one out of every seven) working-age Americans who do not have health insurance?[1] If they were to gain health insurance coverage, would their health improve? This report of the Institute of Medicine (IOM) Committee on the Consequences of Uninsurance addresses these two questions with a critical review and assessment of research that has examined the question of how health insurance affects a range of health-related outcomes for adults.[2]

The Committee is charged with consolidating and critically appraising the evidence regarding the health, social, and economic impacts of uninsurance for individuals, families, communities, and the nation. In this, its second report, the Committee examines the effects on adults' health of lacking coverage by conducting a systematic review of clinical and epidemiological literature that address this question. Finally, the Committee applies its findings from this review to reach conclusions about the likely impact that health insurance would have on the health of uninsured adults.

A critical question for public policy concerning health insurance coverage and the financing of health care more generally is whether health insurance improves personal health outcomes. It is not, however, the only consideration that is rel-

---

[1] See the introductory section of Chapter 4 for a brief description of the social and demographic characteristics of uninsured adults.

[2] The Committee's review primarily focused on adults under age 65 and excluded studies that dealt exclusively with those over 65.

evant to devising fair and compassionate public policies for health insurance and health care programs. Health insurance serves the dual purpose of promoting health by making routine health care services financially accessible and protecting individuals and families against large financial losses in the case of major illness or injury. Public policy recognizes both functions of health insurance in the direct governmental financing of Medicare, Medicaid, and the State Children's Health Insurance Program and indirectly through the federal and state tax subsidies of employment-sponsored health insurance (IOM, 2001a).[3]

This report addresses the first purpose of health insurance only, the effectiveness of insurance coverage in promoting health among those covered. Most of us take for granted that medical services improve our health by relieving pain, reducing functional impairments, curing disease, treating chronic conditions, and making available preventive measures that help us avoid becoming sick or that detect disease at early and readily treatable stages. Even if medical care were not effective in achieving all of these goals, contact with a physician or another health care provider when we are ill or injured, in pain, or not able to function well in everyday life may comfort and reassure us. Health insurance affords us these less tangible but widely appreciated benefits of our interactions with health care providers and institutions. Finally, Americans value health care highly, as evidenced by the large share of the Gross Domestic Product—14 percent—that we devote to it (IOM, 2001a). Most Americans believe that essential care should be and is, in fact, provided to those who need it, regardless of a person's financial resources or health insurance status (IOM, 2001a).

The questions that this report attempts to answer are simple and direct. The evidence that bears on these questions, however, is complex and requires thorough analysis and careful interpretation. If health insurance is found to have a positive effect on personal health, it almost certainly must do so because medical care—the services and access to a health care provider that are paid for and facilitated by health insurance—positively affects one's health. If research does not confirm that health insurance improves personal health however, it does not necessarily mean that medical care is not effective in improving health. Having insurance is neither a necessary nor a sufficient intermediate step in obtaining medical care. Other factors that enhance or diminish personal health, such as educational attainment, family income and disabilities are correlated with different forms of health insurance and may obscure any effects of health insurance on health outcomes. These factors that affect health status and their interactions with health insurance are discussed in Chapters 2 and 4 of this report.

Studies of the impact of health insurance status (that is, whether or not one

---

[3]As discussed in the Committee's previous report, *Coverage Matters*, the value of this tax subsidy increases with income and thus disproportionately benefits higher-income households (IOM, 2001a). This may contribute to the disparity in health insurance coverage rates between higher and lower income groups.

has coverage and, if so, what kind of coverage) on health care and health must take a wide variety of personal and environmental factors into account in order to isolate the effect of coverage. Before presenting findings, the Committee introduces its conceptual framework for identifying these factors and effects related to health insurance coverage, and describes the approach to collecting, evaluating, and interpreting clinical and population survey research. The remainder of this introductory chapter describes the scope of the report, provides basic definitions and classification criteria, and presents the Committee's conceptual framework.

SCOPE OF THE REPORT

This report examines the quantifiable effects, for adults of working age (18 to 65), of having or lacking health insurance on measures of health status (including self-reported health and functioning, mortality, and condition-specific morbidity indicators such as blood pressure for hypertension and blood glucose levels for diabetes) and on measures of the quality and processes of health care. The Committee addresses children's health and health care utilization and perinatal care and outcomes in a forthcoming report that examines them within the dynamic context of the family and of family-level effects of uninsurance. This report also excludes studies limited to people 65 years and older because virtually all elderly have Medicare or comparable insurance coverage.[4]

The health-related effects for adults who lack any form of health insurance are the primary focus of this report. The scope of health insurance benefit packages and service exclusions (for example, whether and the extent to which a health plan covers prescription drugs, mental health services, or screening services) is a secondary focus that emerged in the course of the Committee's review. Studies that compared uninsured adults with those who had various forms of coverage with different benefits, health care utilization, and outcomes had findings that appeared to depend in part on the nature of the benefit package. Furthermore, in a few instances, studies explicitly compared health plans' benefit structures (for example, in the cases of preventive services and mental health care, as discussed in Chapter 3). Thus, the Committee's findings and conclusions reflect the evidence available about the effects of particular benefits and health plan characteristics and compare these for insured and uninsured persons.

Last, this report considers only *health-related* outcomes associated with health insurance status. It does not address the financial impacts on individuals and families of having or lacking coverage, impacts on health care providers and institutions, or societal economic costs. These impacts will each be considered in subsequent Committee reports.

---

[4]While Medicare covers hospitalizations, physician and other outpatient services, including rehabilitative therapies and home health care, it does not cover most outpatient prescription drugs nor does it cover nonrehabilitative long-term care.

DEFINITIONS

The Committee's definitions of *health insurance* and *uninsured* are consistent with those adopted in its previous report, *Coverage Matters: Insurance and Health Care,* reflecting both a policy focus on people who lack any form of financial coverage for basic hospital and physician care and the practical limitations of how information about health insurance status is presented in health services research. "Health insurance" is defined by the Committee as financial coverage for basic hospital and ambulatory care services provided through employment-based indemnity, service-benefit, or managed care plans; individually purchased health insurance policies; public programs such as Medicare, Medicaid and the State Children's Health Insurance Program, and other state-sponsored health plans for specified populations.[5] "Uninsured" refers to persons without *any* form of public or private coverage for hospital and outpatient care for any length of time. The Committee did not set out to examine specific insurance benefits or levels of cost sharing, both of which are relevant to questions about the adequacy of health insurance coverage, or "underinsurance."[6] As discussed immediately above, the research results dictated that the Committee consider evidence and findings related to the scope of benefits covered by various health insurance plans and programs.

Durations of time are important in measuring both health insurance coverage and its effects. Virtually all studies in this field have limitations with respect to measuring periods of coverage and changes in insurance status over time. Studies usually report health insurance status at the time of initial contact with the health care system and enrollment in the study. Any exception to this practice is noted in the discussion of a particular study. Surveys that measure health insurance coverage rates for populations may use any of the following definitions of uninsured:

- uninsured at the time of the interview,
- uninsured that month, or
- uninsured over a past period of a given length (e.g., uninsured for the entire previous year).[7]

---

[5]CHAMPUS, now TriCare, the health insurance program for dependents of active and retired military personnel is classified in some studies as employment-based coverage, and grouped with private plans, and in others (less commonly) as public insurance, and grouped with Medicaid and Medicare. The Committee does not classify Department of Veterans Affairs (VA) health care as health insurance because it provides direct health care to veterans entitled on the basis of disability and serves as a provider of last resort for other veterans. Studies evaluating health insurance status effects most commonly classify VA health care as a separate category or exclude it in recognition of its unique features. Some studies include persons served by VA facilities as publicly insured.

[6]See the Committee's first report, *Coverage Matters* (pp. 27–28) for a brief discussion of underinsurance.

[7]See Appendix B of *Coverage Matters* (IOM, 2001a), for a description of the largest and most frequently cited surveys of health insurance coverage.

The majority of published research literature consists of *cross-sectional analyses* (i.e., studies comparing different groups at a single point in time) that have limited usefulness in understanding the effects of health insurance status longitudinally or over time (e.g., whether health outcomes differ for persons who lack coverage for 6 months compared with those who lack coverage for 18 months), or the effects of transitions or interruptions in coverage over time.

This report uses the terms *needed* or *necessary health care, appropriate health care,* and, less frequently, *guideline-concordant care* to refer to health care and medical services that, with reference to some explicit professional consensus- or evidence-based utilization or practice guidelines, are considered effective and necessary, not only to treat emergency and acute conditions but also to manage chronic disease and sustain or enhance health in those who are well. As discussed in the following section, the Committee has focused its evaluation of the evidence about health insurance on those studies that have used explicit criteria for the appropriate use of health care services.

A CONCEPTUAL FRAMEWORK FOR UNDERSTANDING THE EFFECTS OF HEALTH INSURANCE STATUS

Measuring the unique, or independent, effect of having or lacking health insurance is difficult at best, because investigations of this question are not conducted as randomized, controlled experiments, as are studies of the effect of a drug at a given dosage. Unlike clinical studies of the efficacy of a particular therapeutic intervention (e.g. aspirin after myocardial infarction), studies of the effects of health insurance on health-related outcomes do not randomly assign participants to experimental and control groups, where one group receives the "therapeutic intervention" of health insurance and the other group is denied coverage. Research ethics, over and above practical considerations, preclude this kind of prospective, experimental design in which benefits are withheld.[8]

Furthermore, health insurance or its absence is a characteristic that is closely intertwined with other features of individuals and population groups and with their physical and social environments. Specifically, it is intertwined with the very characteristics—namely, education, income, employment and health status—that influence health insurance coverage (IOM, 2001a). Thus, it is impossible to ad-

---

[8]The notable exception to this generalization is the RAND Health Insurance Experiment, conducted between 1974 and 1982, which randomly assigned roughly 2,000 families in six different sites to one of 14 experimental health insurance plans that varied in their cost-sharing arrangements. Cost sharing ranged from none in the free care plan to 95 percent for all health services, limited to a maximum of $1,000 per family per year (in then-current dollars) with reduced amounts for low-income families (Keeler et al., 1985; Newhouse et al., 1993). The study was designed so that no participating family could be made worse off as a result of their participation than they would have been if they had not participated. This social experiment did not, however, include a study group without any health insurance at all.

minister and measure a "pure" dose of health insurance (and nothing else) and difficult to isolate its effect.

The conceptual framework introduced in the Committee's previous report is adapted here to highlight and explicate the mechanisms by which health insurance influences the kind of health care received and health outcomes. Appendix A presents the Committee's general conceptual framework that was introduced in *Coverage Matters* (IOM, 2001a) as additional background to the discussion here. Figure 1.1 expands the relevant sections of the general framework and focuses on the relationship between health insurance status, the process of obtaining health care, and personal health-related outcomes.

Coverage serves as a means to the end of obtaining services that may induce physiological (and other kinds of) changes that are reflected in various measures of health. Having health insurance does not affect one's health by eliciting a measurable physiological response in those who possess it except, perhaps, by reducing stress and worry about covering medical expenses.[9] *Intermediate measures* of the effect of health insurance on health, and thus mediating factors, include

- having a regular or usual source of care,
- the receipt of "appropriate care," as validated by professional opinion and clinical effectiveness research, and
- the quality of care received.

Health insurance plays both a critical and, at the same time, partial role in facilitating the receipt of appropriate, high-quality health care (Bindman et al., 1996; Eisenberg and Power, 2000). Because many characteristics other than health insurance status (including genetic factors, education, income, social class, personal health practices, beliefs about health care, and social and physical environment) affect the ultimate outcome of interest—health status—directly, intermediate measures are often used as proxies for health outcomes in studies of health insurance effects. These intermediate measures are represented by the boxes entitled "Process of Care" and "Intermediate Outcomes" in Figure 1.1.

The Committee considers both intermediate measures and final health outcomes as *health-related outcomes* to determine the impact of health insurance status on personal health. *Health-related outcomes* include self-reported overall health status and measures of evaluated health such as mortality, functional status, disability, stage of disease at the time of diagnosis, and a number of condition-specific physiological and behavioral indicators, such as blood pressure control for hypertension and blood glucose levels for diabetes.[10] Figure 1.1 also includes a commu-

---

[9]There is a research literature on the relationship between psychological stress and healing; see Kiecolt-Glaser et al. (1998) for a description of the theory and evidence.

[10]Household or general population health surveys often include questions about participants' overall health status. These subjective measures have been validated as corresponding well to health outcomes such as mortality (Mossey and Shapiro, 1982; Idler et al., 1990; Franks et al., 1993b).

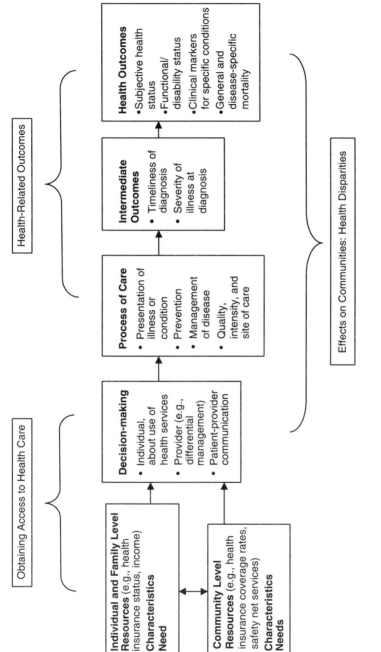

FIGURE 1.1 A conceptual framework for assessing the effect of health insurance status on health-related outcomes for adults.

nity-level outcome, which emerged as an important finding in the course of conducting the research literature review, namely, the impact of health insurance on the extent of health disparities among racial and ethnic population groups.

The Committee considers measures of the process of health care delivery, such as quality of care and the number or frequency of health care services, as health-related outcomes only if they have been endorsed as widely recognized professional guidelines or validated by science-based effectiveness studies as determinative of final health outcomes. For example, the recommendations of the U.S. Preventive Health Services Task Force regarding the frequency of Pap smears to detect cervical cancer establish the appropriateness criterion that the Committee uses in evaluating evidence from studies that compare the receipt of cervical cancer screening by insured and uninsured women. (See Box 3.2 in Chapter 3.) It is important to look at intermediate health outcomes such as receipt of cancer screening tests at the recommended intervals because many final health outcomes (e.g., diagnosed cancer or death) are not evident or realized for many years and very few studies of health insurance status extend over a long enough time to capture these outcomes.

ORGANIZATION OF THE REPORT

The Committee's critical assessment of the research literature is described, its findings are presented, and the implications of its findings and conclusions are discussed in the remaining chapters of this report.

Chapter 2 outlines the report's analytic design and methods. First, it details the Committee's conceptualization of how health insurance status affects access to health care services, which in turn affects health outcomes. Next it identifies important covariates of health insurance, such as health status, race and ethnicity, and socioeconomic status and considers analytic approaches to disentangling their effects on health-related outcomes.

Chapter 3 presents the Committee's findings based on its literature review. These findings are summarized within categories that reflect both type of service (e.g., preventive services, disease management for chronic conditions, hospital-based care) and condition-specific outcomes (e.g., stage of disease at detection and mortality rates for cancers), in addition to overall measures of health and mortality for large population samples.

Chapter 4 employs the findings enumerated in Chapter 3 to draw conclusions about the effects of coverage on health outcomes for specific population groups that are at particular risk of adverse effects from lacking coverage and about the features of health insurance that account for its effects on health outcomes. Last, the Committee considers the potential benefits of extending health insurance to the U.S. population of uninsured adults.

2

Mechanisms and Methods: Looking At the Impact of Health Insurance on Health

The relationships between health insurance and access to health care, and health insurance and care received, have been the subject of hundreds of studies over the past several decades. More recently, the relationship between health insurance and health outcomes has also been examined. This chapter describes the Committee's analytic approach to its critical review of this research to inform the understanding of the relationships between health insurance, health care, and health outcomes for adults.

The chapter is organized in three sections. First, it outlines the mechanisms by which the Committee postulates that health insurance affects health-related outcomes. Whether one has health insurance, a regular source of care and, if one is uninsured, the length of time that one is without coverage all influence access to care and affect health-related outcomes.

The second section discusses issues related to the measurement of health insurance effects and considerations of research design that affect the inferences that can be drawn. It explores analytic strategies to distinguish the effects of health insurance status from those of personal attributes that are correlated with health insurance, including health status, race and ethnicity, and socioeconomic status, which may confound[1] the results of studies that relate health insurance to health outcomes. The section gives particular attention to the two-way causal relationship between health status and insurance status.[2] It also describes the major popu-

---

[1]See Appendix C for definitions of technical terms such as "confound."

[2]Perhaps most problematic for determining the effects of health insurance on personal health is that an individual's health condition may be directly related to enrollment in particular kinds of insurance

lation surveys and databases that provide information about Americans' use of health care and epidemiological information about health status and disease prevalence. These sources provide the data for many of the most informative studies reviewed.

The final section of this chapter presents the Committee's methods for systematic review and synthesis of the research on health insurance status effects. This section describes how studies were identified for inclusion in the review, the criteria for evaluating the methodological quality of studies and study results, and how the Committee's findings are presented in Chapter 3.

MECHANISMS AND MEASURES OF ACCESS TO HEALTH CARE

Health insurance facilitates access to health care by removing or diminishing financial barriers to obtaining care. Among people who have insurance, the extent of cost sharing also influences the use of health care (Newhouse et al., 1993; Zweifel and Manning, 2000). An extensive body of research consistently finds a strong and positive relationship between health insurance and access to care, even as the definitions and measures of access have been strengthened. Population-based surveys conducted over the past three decades have evaluated access to primary care in relation to health insurance status with measures such as any physician visit within a year, the number of physician visits per year, having a regular source of care, and the ability to obtain care when needed (Freeman and Corey, 1993; Hafner-Eaton, 1993; Newacheck et al., 1998; Nelson et al., 1999; Zuvekas and Weinick, 1999; Haley and Zuckerman, 2000; Kasper et al., 2000; Shi, 2000; Weinick et al., 2000; Hoffman et al., 2001).

Public policy and health care industry interests in high-quality and efficient health care have developed in tandem with the progress of clinical effectiveness research over the past decade. The standards of evidence for the efficacy of health insurance in promoting better health outcomes have evolved from enumerating physician visits to measurable improvements in effective processes of care. The notion of "access" itself has shifted from a simple measure of utilization to measures that incorporate the quality of care and health outcomes. In 1993, the Institute of Medicine (IOM) Committee on Monitoring Access to Personal Health Care Services reconceptualized access as "the timely use of personal health services to achieve the best possible health outcomes" and recommended a set of health outcome measures that could serve to monitor populations over time for access to basic health services (Millman, 1993).

---

programs (e.g., as a medically needy or disabled Medicaid beneficiary and other Medicaid enrollees who join the program only when they incur a hospitalization or need other expensive care; in the case of nongroup private health insurance, only persons in good health may be accepted for coverage). See Box 2-1 for further discussion.

In studies of access to care and health outcomes, several factors mediate the relationship between health insurance and health-related outcomes. These include being able to see a provider when one believes care is needed, having a regular source of health care, having continuity of coverage, and the duration of periods without health insurance. Measures for each of these factors provide some information about an individual's or population's access to health services that supplements the measurement of health insurance status at a given point in time. These measures are discussed below.

Getting Care When Needed

The ability to see a physician or other health care provider when one believes medical attention is needed is a fundamental and intuitive measure of access to health care. Most Americans mistakenly believe that people without health insurance have this level of access (IOM, 2001a). Although the lack of health insurance is not the only reason someone might not be able to see a health care practitioner when needed, it is a major one.[3] Adults without health insurance are far more likely to go without health care that they believe they need than are adults with health insurance of any kind (Lurie et al., 1984, 1986; Berk and Schur, 1998; Burstin et al., 1998; Baker et al., 2000; Kasper et al., 2000; Schoen and DesRoches, 2000; Davidoff et al., 2001; Holahan and Spillman, 2002).

While the *overall* percentage of adults who reported that cost prevented them from seeing a doctor in the previous 12 months increased only slightly from 10 percent to 11 percent between 1991 and 1996, the proportion of *uninsured* adults who reported this barrier to care increased from 28 to 35 percent, and the fraction of insured adults reporting this barrier decreased slightly from 8 to 7 percent (Nelson et al., 1999).[4] In 1998, nearly 70 percent of uninsured adults in poor health could not see a doctor at some time during the year because of cost (Ayanian et al., 2000). A study that polled 1,100 patients four months after their initial visit to an emergency department found that patients who lost their health insurance were more than twice as likely as those who maintained their coverage to have delayed seeking care in the four-month interval (Burstin et al., 1998).

Evaluations based on professional judgment confirm findings based on a subjectively determined need for care. In one study with a national probability sample of almost 3,500 adult respondents, a physician panel identified 15 serious conditions for which they deemed medical attention necessary (Baker et al., 2000). In

---

[3]Other reasons include not being able to find a provider within traveling distance and not being able to find a practitioner that participates in one's health plan (particularly a problem for Medicaid enrollees in states with low provider payment levels), language or cultural barriers, and understanding of symptoms and health conditions as requiring professional attention. See the IOM report, *Access to Health Care in America* (Millman, 1993) for a discussion of barriers to access.

[4]All of these differences are statistically significant.

an analysis that adjusted for demographic and economic characteristics and also for health status and having a regular source of care, the authors found that an uninsured adult was much less likely than an insured adult to get care for a reported symptom (odds ratio [OR] = 0.43). Examining only those symptoms for which the respondent thought care was needed, those without insurance were even less likely to have received care (OR = 0.28). Among those who did not receive needed care, the uninsured were far more likely than those with insurance to report that they did not get care because of cost (95 percent and 23 percent, respectively) (Baker et al., 2000).[5]

A lack of health insurance acts not only as an initial barrier to care but may continue to impede the receipt of appropriate, effective care. Even if uninsured patients receive primary care, referrals to specialists, ancillary diagnostic and treatment services and medications are more difficult to obtain. Primary care providers who treat uninsured and other low-income patients report greater difficulty in arranging for referrals and services that they cannot directly provide for their uninsured patients than for those who are insured (Fairbrother et al., 2002).

Persons who never present themselves to a health care provider are not accounted for in health services research that documents and measures utilization and outcomes with hospital administrative records, patient chart reviews, and clinic encounter forms. This is a "blind spot" and source of bias in studies of health insurance effects because overall, persons without health insurance are estimated to use roughly two-thirds of the services that those who do have insurance use (Marquis and Long, 1995). Because those without health insurance are less likely to see a provider than are others with insurance and thus are less likely to be included in research documentation, studies that rely on health care records to compare groups who received some care may overstate utilization by uninsured populations.

Having a Regular Source of Care

In addition to supplying the financial resources that enable one to obtain health care when needed, insurance coverage also improves receipt of appropriate care by facilitating the use of a regular source of care or primary care provider.[6]

---

[5]Previously reported in IOM (2001a).

[6]Measurement of a usual or regular source of care is frequently based on survey participant responses to a single question such as "Is there a place or health care practitioner that you routinely go to for medical care?" However, some studies use more restrictive definitions of a regular source of care (e.g., they exclude hospital emergency departments as a positive response to the question.) The studies included in this review that document a regular source of care may use different operational definitions. One problem with evaluating utilization outcomes in terms of having a regular source of care is that frequent users of services are more likely to report having a regular source; the direction of causality is not clear. As the concept of primary care has been further conceptualized, the attributes associated with a regular source of care have become more specific (Starfield, 1992, 1998; Shi, 2000).

Both health insurance and having a regular source of care contribute independently to the utilization of health services (Solis et al., 1990; Mosen et al, 1998; Mandelblatt et al., 1999; Zuvekas and Weinick, 1999; Cummings et al., 2000; Breen et al. 2001). Having a regular source of care enhances the appropriate use of ambulatory care as measured by receipt of preventive services, management of chronic conditions, and population rates of avoidable hospitalizations (Bindman et al., 1995; Starfield, 1995; Pappas et al., 1997; Kozak et al., 2001).

The independent contribution that having a regular source of care makes to the receipt of appropriate care reinforces rather than diminishes the importance of health insurance, because health insurance is an important determinant of obtaining and maintaining an ongoing relationship with a health care provider. Adults with health insurance are much more likely than those who are uninsured to have a regular source of care, a consistent finding across states with very different health care resources and provider configurations (IOM, 2001a; Holahan and Spillman, 2002). An analysis based on the 1997 National Health Interview Survey found that among adults eligible for Medicaid, 42 percent of those not enrolled in the program did not have a regular source of care, whereas only 12 percent of those with Medicaid coverage lacked one (Davidoff et al., 2001). Even those uninsured adults who have chronic conditions are substantially more likely to lack a regular source of care than are chronically ill adults with health insurance. Among uninsured adults, 19 percent with heart disease, 14 percent with hypertension, and 26 percent with arthritis do not have a regular source of care, compared with 8, 4, and 7 percent, respectively, of their insured counterparts (Fish-Parcham, 2001).

Someone without health insurance who can identify a regular source of care may still face difficulties in obtaining recommended and effective health care services that are outside the scope of practice of their regular provider, such as referrals to specialists, ancillary services, and hospital-based care.

Continuity of Care and Coverage

Not only is continuity of *care*, as measured by having a regular source of care, important, continuity of insurance *coverage* is also critical to the receipt of appropriate care. Breaks in coverage can disrupt care relationships to the detriment of quality health care. Being uninsured for longer periods of time can be expected to have larger effects on utilization of services (and consequently on health) than being uninsured for shorter periods. Although only a few studies have examined health outcomes by length of time uninsured (Lurie et al., 1984, 1986; Ayanian et al., 2000; Kasper et al., 2000; Baker et al., 2001), a number of studies have looked at intermediate measures of access to care and volume of services (e.g., any physician visit or number of visits within a year) and find strong relationships between breaks in coverage and length of time uninsured, on the one hand, and reduced access to and utilization of services, on the other (Burstin et al, 1998;

Ayanian et al., 2000; Kasper et al., 2000; Schoen and DesRoches, 2000; Hoffman et al., 2001).[7]

One study examined clinical outcomes in a small cohort of patients with high blood pressure who were followed after some of them lost Medi-Cal coverage (California's Medicaid program). Blood pressure control for those who lost public insurance was worse at six months than at one year following the loss of coverage. The authors hypothesize that the deterioration in blood pressure control was reversed to some extent after new care arrangements were established following the termination of benefits (Lurie et al., 1986). In another study that compared transitions among health care plans to the complete loss of coverage, researchers found evidence of a temporary weakening of access to care among those who *changed* plans and a more pronounced loss of access among those who *lost* health insurance (Burstin et al., 1998). The experience of intermittently insured adults, in terms of both access and outcome measures, falls between that of continuously insured adults and continuously uninsured adults but is more similar to the latter than the former (Schoen and DesRoches, 2000; Baker et al., 2001). These results suggest that continuity and stability in health insurance coverage contribute to reliable access and effective health care.

Finally, in a large-scale survey comparing persons uninsured for shorter or longer time periods, measures of access, appropriate care, and health status were worse for those uninsured for longer periods (Ayanian et al., 2000). These findings are particularly relevant to the interpretation of results for Medicaid enrollees, whose coverage tends to be of limited duration and who may have been uninsured before they were enrolled in Medicaid (IOM, 2001a; Perkins et al., 2001). In fact, more than half of single women with Medicaid at the beginning of a year have lost their coverage before the end of the year, and between one-third and one-half of them are uninsured a year after they lose Medicaid coverage (Short and Freedman, 1998; Garrett and Holahan, 2000).

METHODOLOGY AND MEASUREMENT OF HEALTH INSURANCE EFFECTS

Chapter 1 poses the problem of how to determine whether a "dose" of health insurance is effective in improving an individual's health. Experimental studies provide a stronger research design than observational studies for concluding that insurance itself affects health. However, most of the research examining the impact of health insurance on health-related outcomes is based on observational

---

[7]Although access to health care services measured at this most general level (i.e., in terms of the number of visits to physicians and self-reported delays in seeking care) is not the focus of the Committee's review, it can be postulated that longer times without coverage that result in more greatly reduced utilization and delayed care would similarly affect the specific health-related outcomes examined in this report.

(nonexperimental) and, with several important exceptions, cross-sectional (point-in-time, nonlongitudinal) studies. Indeed, earlier reviews of the research on health insurance status and health outcomes have highlighted the need for longitudinal studies and close examination of natural experiments, for example, when public coverage programs are expanded to new population groups or cut back or among state-level programs with differing eligibility standards (Weissman and Epstein, 1994; Brown et al., 1998). The one major randomized trial of health insurance, the RAND Health Insurance Experiment, did not have an uninsured group, although it did include a group with 95 percent cost sharing and a very high deductible, which approximated no coverage for routine care (Newhouse et al., 1993).[8]

Because of the great potential for biases in observational studies, the associations observed between health insurance status and health may reflect the effects of factors other than health insurance, such as income, social status, or education. Much of the observational research, especially that conducted in the past decade, has included extensive statistical adjustment for some of these potentially confounding factors. Such adjustment strengthens the analytic design of observational studies and increases the likelihood that the observed associations between health insurance and health outcomes represent a causal relationship. However, additional, less readily measured personal characteristics covary with health insurance status and may also affect health outcomes.

This section examines the sources of potential bias and the analytic strategies used to address them in observational studies of health insurance effects. It also reviews the personal characteristics that are most likely to covary with health insurance status—namely, health status, race and ethnicity, and socioeconomic status (SES) and considers how they may confound findings of health insurance effects in observational studies. [9]

Limits of Observational Studies

Sources of Bias

In relying on observational studies to determine whether and how health insurance affects health-related outcomes, the first limitation is the wide variability

---

[8]See footnote 8 in Chapter 1.

[9]See the Committee's earlier report, *Coverage Matters*, for an analysis of personal characteristics related to health insurance (IOM, 2001a). In this report "race–ethnicity" is used to refer to the classification of population groups according to U.S. Census categories unless otherwise indicated. "Socioeconomic status" encompasses a variety of indicators, including income, educational attainment, type of employment or job classification, and residential area. Health insurance status itself has often been used as a measure of SES. Most studies of health insurance status effects include at most two or three SES indicators in addition to race–ethnicity as control variables.

in how the term "health insurance" is defined and measured. In cross-sectional studies, a participant's health insurance status is measured at one point in time, when other personal information is collected or when health care services are used and utilization is documented in administrative or clinical records. Even longitudinal studies that follow a study participant across time often measure health insurance status only at the beginning of the study period. Because health insurance status may change over time (with the important exception of those who qualify, on any basis, for Medicare), the classification of study participants as "insured" includes not only those who always had insurance, but also those who may have recently been uninsured and now have coverage. Likewise, those classified as uninsured include not only those who have always been without health insurance, but also those who may have had coverage until recently. The result of the point-in-time measurement of health insurance status is to diminish the ability to measure any effect of health insurance on health outcomes because the groups being compared have overlapping membership. Therefore, the actual effect of health insurance, if it were to be measured in terms of its duration, may be greater than found in observational studies that look at insurance status at a single point in time.

Most studies of health insurance effects do not fully account for a second kind of bias in measuring health insurance coverage, namely, the wide range of benefit packages and of cost-sharing and provider participation arrangements subsumed under the category of general health insurance. Health insurance plans that cover a wide array of benefits or that require no or limited cost sharing (deductibles and coinsurance) from enrollees can be expected to affect patient and provider behavior differently from plans that cover fewer benefits and require more cost sharing (Zweifel and Manning, 2000). Finally, health insurance plans differ in terms of provider payment and participation rates and arrangements, affecting enrollees' ease of access to care and patterns of utilization.

Another potential source of bias in observational studies is the nonrandom distribution or selection of study participants among health insurance status categories. Health status is itself a determinant of health insurance coverage. It is closely related to the likelihood that someone has insurance and to the kind of coverage he or she has (IOM, 2001a). Working-age adults in better health are more likely to work full time and at higher paying jobs, thus increasing their chances of having employment-based health insurance. At the same time, those with access to employment-based coverage who anticipate needing health care are somewhat more likely to take up the offer of coverage than similar persons in good health with no expectation of significant health care use and expense. Adults in poor health without access to employment-based coverage are more likely to seek individually purchased coverage but may find that they cannot obtain health insurance because of preexisting conditions. Those in the poorest health who are unable to work (i.e., who are recognized as permanently and totally disabled) or who have very low incomes or high medical expenses may qualify for Medicare or Medicaid. Box 2-1 reviews the eligibility requirements for Medicaid and Medicare that contribute to the distinctive health status profile of working-age adults with public health insurance.

Thus, health status differs systematically among persons grouped by health insurance categories because health status is one criterion by which people qualify for coverage, and analytic adjustments for underlying health status tend to be incomplete at best. Health-related behaviors such as smoking, exercise, and diet also affect individual health and are sometimes but not usually included as covariates in analyses of health insurance effects.[10] These health behaviors are strongly related to educational attainment, which itself is correlated with health insurance status (IOM, 2001a). Finally, additional personal characteristics, such as the willingness to live with risk and the value placed on good health or health care, may bias the selection of enrollees in private health insurance plans, including those who take up the offer of employment-based coverage and those who seek to purchase individual coverage. Because most of those offered employment-based coverage do accept it and relatively few purchase individual coverage, this source of selection bias is not likely to substantially affect the overall comparisons between insured and uninsured adults.

Major Covariates

Personal characteristics that vary with health insurance status may confound analyses of the effects of health insurance on health-related outcomes because they are independently associated with these outcomes. In addition to health status, which has just been discussed, the most important among these characteristics are race and ethnicity and SES. Race and ethnicity are frequently included in analyses that examine the effects of health insurance status on health outcomes. SES, however, is more difficult to separate completely from health insurance status, even when it is represented in multivariable statistical analyses by employment, educational attainment, or income. In addition, distinctive ethnic and cultural population groups with different economic and behavioral characteristics are subsumed under the broad racial and ethnic categories most commonly used in research. For example, Mexican and Cuban Americans and Puerto Ricans are all categorized as Hispanic; likewise, African and Caribbean immigrants may be categorized with African Americans as Black.

Racial and ethnic minority groups and persons with lower SES often face barriers to obtaining health care, such as lack of transportation, concerns with personal safety, and provider shortages, that extend beyond those related to being uninsured. Even with insurance and health care, disadvantaged groups often have worse health on average than do socially privileged groups.

---

[10]See the report *Promoting Health: Intervention Strategies from Social and Behavioral Research*, (IOM, 2000b) for a review and analysis of behavioral factors in health.

BOX 2.1
Health Insurance and Health Status

The average health status of adults with private (employment-sponsored or individually purchased) health insurance and those with public health insurance differs, and both differ from the average health status of uninsured adults. Taken together, adults under age 65 with private health insurance are healthier than adults without any insurance, who are in turn healthier than adults with public insurance (Sorlie et al., 1994; Hahn and Flood, 1995).

Privately Insured Adults

Both adults who have employment-sponsored group insurance and those who have individually purchased policies have better-than-average health status. In the case of employment-sponsored group coverage, insured adults either are working or are the dependents of workers. Workers have a better health status than nonworkers, and insured workers have higher family incomes than uninsured workers. Adults with individual coverage (e.g., the self-employed and early retirees) face health screening and risk-rated premiums, and thus tend to be both healthier and wealthier than counterparts who do not obtain individual coverage.

Publicly Insured Adults

Adults under age 65 obtain health coverage from a public program, either Medicare or Medicaid, because they are sick, poor, or medically needy. Adults with public program coverage tend to be in substantially worse health than those with private insurance and in somewhat worse health than uninsured adults.

Medicare includes people under 65 who have been covered by the Social Se-

Rates of health insurance coverage differ for various racial and ethnic groups: African Americans, Asian Americans and Pacific Islanders, and Hispanics are much more likely to be uninsured than are non-Hispanic whites. Eighteen and a half (18.5) percent of African Americans, 18 percent of Asian Americans and Pacific Islanders, and 32 percent of Hispanics are uninsured, compared with 10 percent of whites (Mills, 2001). Ethnic differences in insurance status partially reflect differences in the rates of employment-sponsored insurance coverage. Public insurance programs (e.g., Medicaid) only partially make up for these disparities in employment-sponsored coverage (Gabel, 1999; Monheit and Vistnes, 2000; IOM, 2001a).

Insurance is also correlated with socioeconomic status. Forty (40) percent of adults who live in lower-income families (defined as having incomes less than 200 percent of the federal poverty level and 40 percent of adults without a high school diploma are uninsured, compared with 10 percent of adults with at least a college degree (Hoffman and Pohl, 2000; Monheit and Vistnes, 2000).

In addition, the factors of race–ethnicity and SES are intertwined. In the United States, ethnic minorities face more limited educational and occupational opportunities. Many ethnic minorities live in highly segregated communities (Massey and Denton, 1989; Cutler et al., 1999). These neighborhoods may be

curity Disability Insurance program for at least two years and those certified as having end-stage renal disease.

Medicaid eligibility is based on income and on additional categorical criteria, such as being pregnant, being disabled or blind, or being a parent with dependent children. If others with incomes higher than the state Medicaid eligibility limit have sufficiently high medical expenses, they are considered "medically needy" and qualify. In most states, beneficiaries must periodically re-enroll, making periods without insurance relatively common. The median length of time that an adult under age 65 remains on Medicaid is 5 months (Tin and Castro, 2001). There is a greater likelihood that a Medicaid enrollee has just been or is about to become uninsured than is the case for privately insured individuals. Last, many eligible people do not enroll until they seek medical care and the hospital or clinic signs them up in order to receive payment for services provided (Davidoff et al., 2001). Thus, the healthier among those eligible for Medicaid are less likely to be enrolled than those who are sicker.

Uninsured Adults

Some adults who are uninsured are eligible for Medicaid but not enrolled. Adults who meet income and other eligibility standards may not feel the need to enroll if they do not have unmet health care needs. These adults who are eligible but not enrolled in Medicaid have better overall health status and fewer activity limitations or chronic conditions than otherwise comparable adults enrolled in Medicaid. Since the enactment of federal welfare legislation in 1996, some adults have mistakenly believed that they are not eligible (Garrett and Holahan, 2000). Other uninsured adults with social and economic characteristics similar to those of persons enrolled in Medicaid do not meet other eligibility requirements.

more crowded, offer fewer economic opportunities, be more geographically isolated from health care providers, and have more environmental health hazards. Each of these factors may adversely affect health. Boxes 2.2 and 2.3 illustrate how health insurance is just one of several sources of health disparities among racial and ethnic groups and persons of different SES.

Context of Care

Every study that examines the care and outcomes for people without health insurance does so within a particular economic and institutional context of health care for the dominant population, namely, those with health insurance. Nationally, one out of every six or seven adults receiving health care is uninsured. Among states, the ratio of uninsured to insured ranges from one in ten (Minnesota and Rhode Island) to one in four (Texas, Arizona, New Mexico) (IOM, 2001a). Two points follow from this observation. First, national studies that examine the health care and outcomes of uninsured adults mask a wide range of health care financing contexts within which care is rendered. Second, any evaluation of the care of uninsured adults reflects the financing and resource environment that

BOX 2.2
Race and Ethnicity

The effect of race and ethnicity on access to care and health outcomes operates through a number of mechanisms, many not directly linked to financial barriers or health insurance status. Some of the racial and ethnic differences in mortality are reflected in differences in the prevalence of specific illnesses and events, such as cancer, cardiovascular disease, substance use, diabetes, infant mortality, and homicide. Even when mortality rates are adjusted to reflect both the prevalence of these conditions and for income, however, one-third of the difference in the mortality rate between blacks and whites remains (Mutchler and Burr, 1991). Some have suggested that racial and ethnic differences in health are due largely to differences in SES (Sorlie et al., 1994). Yet, at each level of income, African Americans have higher mortality than whites, suggesting that racial and ethnic disparities are not explained solely by differences in socioeconomic status (Pamuk et al., 1998). Last, access to health care may be impeded by language barriers for ethnic minorities, especially but not exclusively among immigrants.

Among Hispanics in the United States a greater degree of acculturation (and thus higher income) appears to be associated with a *decline* in health status (Vega and Amaro, 1994). Since acculturation may be associated with greater educational and employment opportunities, this also suggests that the effect of ethnicity is independent of SES and may be related to social structure, diet, life style, and other health practices and beliefs. Race or ethnicity may be a marker for other cultural beliefs that go beyond the commonly examined labels used in health services research. For example, beliefs about the causes of cancer may differ between African Americans and whites (Maynard et al., 1986).

Cultural differences between patients and providers may result in poor communication that undermines effective care and patients' adherence to treatment regimens (IOM, 2002). Cultural similarity between patients and providers may facilitate communication and decision making (Komaromy et al., 1996; Saha et al., 1999; Schulman et al., 1999). Because African Americans and Hispanics are underrepresented in the health care professions, this concordance is often not realized (Collins et al., 1999; Saha et al., 1999, IOM, 2002).

Racial bias in diagnosis and treatment is yet another potential explanation of the observed disparities (Reisch et al., 2000; IOM, 2002). Further, beyond implicit bias, the experience of overt discrimination may directly affect both access to care and health. Discrimination may affect trust in the patient–doctor relationship, which in turn may also affect the use of health care and health outcomes (Maynard et al, 1986; Doescher et al., 2000). Discrimination may restrict the choice of health care providers, and therefore the quality of care available (Krieger et al., 1993). Finally, the experience of racism may directly result in psychological distress that could adversely affect health (Broman, 1996; Carrasquillo et al., 2000).

prevails at that time and, if the balance of uninsured to insured populations changes, the general processes and outcomes of care may also change, for both those who have and those who lack health insurance. This phenomenon will be addressed in a subsequent Committee report on community impacts of uninsured populations.

BOX 2.3
Socioeconomic Status

SES affects health through a variety of mechanisms. While some of these are directly related to limited financial resources, others are related to health less directly, through belief, behaviors, and environmental factors. Socioeconomic disadvantage can have a continuing or cumulative effect throughout an individual's life. For example, poverty in childhood may affect the health status of an adult (Lynch et al., 1994,1997; Krieger et al., 2001). The relationship between SES and health is bidirectional. In addition to SES influencing health, poor health may cause declines in SES related to loss of employment or income (Adler et al., 1994). This makes the interpretation of cross-sectional studies examining the relationship between SES and health particularly challenging.

Education and income are critical. Low educational attainment, poverty, and economic hardship have each been associated with higher rates of chronic illness, poor self-reported health status, disability, and lower life expectancy (Haan et al., 1987; Pincus et al., 1987; Marmot et al., 1991; Winkleby et al., 1992; Guralnik et al., 1993; Elo and Preston, 1996; Ostrove et al., 2000; van Rossum et al., 2000). Even among those with access to care, individuals with less education may be less able to communicate with their provider, understand risk factors or symptoms of disease, schedule an appointment, or manage their own health condition (Kunst and Mackenbach, 1994; Behera et al., 2000).

Health behaviors such as diet, physical activity, smoking, and alcohol or illicit drug use are also strongly associated with both health outcomes and SES (Otten et al., 1990; Ford et al., 1991; Winkleby et al., 1992; Dixon et al., 2001). A strong inverse association between number of years of education and smoking, cholesterol level, blood pressure, and body mass index exists for the U.S. population (Winkleby et al., 1992). Other potential pathways by which SES may affect health include the following:

- living in neighborhoods with more crowding (with more potential for exposure to communicable diseases), higher rates of violence, and more pollution (Samet et al., 2000);
- greater exposure to stressful life events with associated risk of illness (Cohen et al., 1991; Ruberman et al, 1991); and
- less ability to take time off from work to see the doctor or to arrange for child care or transportation for a visit.

National Surveys and Databases

Many of the studies reviewed draw on a number of publicly sponsored surveys with national or state-level probability samples, epidemiological databases, and disease registries. Box 2.4 identifies these surveys and data sources. The size of these sample surveys, the comprehensiveness of reporting systems, and the collection of comparable data periodically over several years and even decades contribute to the quality of the information available from these sources.

BOX 2.4
Surveys and Databases

Surveys

The **National Health Interview Survey (NHIS)** is a continuous nationwide household interview survey conducted by the National Center for Health Statistics (NCHS). It is designed to allow the development of national estimates of health status and health services utilization of the U.S. civilian noninstitutionalized population. The NHIS has been conducted since 1957, with the core content of the survey being updated approximately every 10–15 years. Interviewers obtain information on personal and demographic characteristics, illnesses, injuries, impairments, chronic conditions, utilization of health services, health insurance, and other topics from about 43,000 households comprising approximately 106,000 individuals.

The **National Health and Nutrition Examination Survey (NHANES)** conducted by the NCHS is designed to assess the health and nutritional status of adults and children in the United States through interviews and direct physical examinations. Approximately 5,000 people are examined each year. NHANES was conducted periodically from 1960 to 1994 with seven national surveys completed during that time. The most recently published data are for the six-year survey conducted between 1988 and 1994, referred to as NHANES III. Since 1999 surveys have been conducted on an annual basis. NHANES collects information on chronic disease prevalence and conditions, risk factors, diet and nutritional status, immunization status, and specific clinical measures such as blood pressure, blood cholesterol, blood sugar, mental health, oral health, and physical functioning.

The **Behavioral Risk Factor Surveillance System (BRFSS)** is an ongoing telephone-based surveillance system designed by the Centers for Disease Control and Prevention (CDC) and conducted separately by each state. Approximately 150,000 adults are interviewed each year. BRFSS monitors modifiable risk behaviors and other factors contributing to the leading causes of morbidity and mortality in the U.S. population. A standardized questionnaire is used to collect information on self-reported health habits and risk factors that contribute to the development of chronic diseases. States participate in the selection of questions that will be asked uniformly across the states. The primary data included in this survey are alcohol and tobacco use, use of preventive health services, HIV/AIDS, health status, limitations of activity, and health care access and utilization.

The **Medical Expenditure Panel Survey (MEPS)**, conducted by the Agency for Healthcare Research and Quality (AHRQ) for the first time in 1996, affords a comprehensive view of national health care utilization, household health expenditures, and health insurance coverage. MEPS consists of four linked, integrated surveys:

1. The Household Component—A sample of families and individuals across the nation, drawn from a subsample of households that participated in the prior year's NHIS. Approximately 13,000 families and 36,000 persons are represented in five interviews conducted over 30 months. Data are collected on health status, health insurance coverage, health care use and expenditures, and sources of payment for health services.

2. Nursing Home Component—A national sample of nursing homes and resi-

dents. Data are collected on the characteristics of facilities and services offered, expenditures and sources of payment by resident, and resident characteristics.

3. Medical Provider Component—A national sample of hospitals, physicians, and home health care providers. Data are gathered to supplement information from the household component and can be used to estimate the expenses of people enrolled in health maintenance organizations and other types of managed care.

4. Insurance Component—Information from the Household Component and from a sample of businesses and government agencies that offer insurance coverage. For the Household Component, data are collected on the health insurance that respondents have had or that has been offered to them. The additional sample consists of data gathered from health plans and health insurance sponsors. This survey is used to develop national, regional, and state-level estimates of the amount, type, and cost of employment-based health insurance.

The **National Medical Expenditure Survey (NMES)** was conducted in 1987 and is a predecessor to MEPS. NMES was a three-part national survey of the U.S. civilian noninstitutionalized population, including surveys of households, medical providers, health plans, and employers. Approximately 13,500 households were surveyed about their demographic background, medical use, costs, and payments.

The **National Medical Care Expenditure Survey (NMCES)**, conducted in 1977, assessed the cost and extent of health insurance in the United States. NMCES included about 14,000 households. It is now known as the National Medical Expenditure Survey-1.

The **Health and Retirement Study (HRS)**, sponsored by the National Institute on Aging and conducted by the University of Michigan, gathers information on the various characteristics of those near or in retirement. It is a longitudinal national panel study that at baseline (1992) sampled 7,600 households with at least one member between the ages of 51 and 61, with follow-ups every 2 years, planned for 12 years. The data collected include economic, demographic, and health information, generally related to retirement issues, for more than 22,000 Americans over the age of 50.

The **Current Population Survey (CPS)** is a nationwide sample survey of about 50,000 households representing 116,000 persons conducted monthly for the Bureau of Labor Statistics by the U.S. Bureau of the Census. It is the primary source of information on the employment characteristics of the U.S. civilian noninstitutionalized population. Since 1980, the CPS has included questions about health insurance coverage along with other demographic characteristics. Both the February and the March supplements to the CPS contain information related to health insurance.

The **HIV Cost and Services Utilization Study (HCSUS)** is a major research effort to collect information on a nationally representative sample of people under care for HIV infection. The HCSUS is funded by AHRQ and conducted by RAND. The original survey (1994–2000) collected data on more than 3,700 HIV-positive people in hospitals, clinics, and private practices in 28 urban and 24 clusters of rural counties. The HCSUS design includes a baseline in-person interview, two follow-up interviews scheduled for 6 months and 12 months after the baseline, and data from patients' medical, pharmaceutical, and billing records.

The HCSUS is composed of a core study and seven supplemental studies. The core study examines cost, use of health services, quality of care, access to and unmet needs for care, quality of life, social support, knowledge of HIV, clinical

BOX 2-4 Continued

outcomes, mental health, and the relationship of these variables to provider type and patient characteristics.

Databases

The **Healthcare Cost and Utilization Project (HCUP)** is a database maintained by AHRQ. HCUP is a partnership among states, the private sector, and the federal government to develop a standardized, multistate health data system on the use of health care services in small areas, the states, and the nation. Currently, 22 states contribute data to the project. HCUP includes a wide array of uniformly formatted administrative databases containing detailed information about hospital inpatients, ambulatory surgeries, and emergency services.

The **Surveillance, Epidemiology, and End Results Program (SEER)** is a comprehensive source of population-based information on cancer incidence and survival data coordinated by the National Cancer Institute. Data are obtained from 11 population-based cancer registries and 3 supplemental registries covering approximately 14 percent of the U.S. population. Information on more than 2.5 million cancer cases is included in the SEER database, and about 160,000 new cases are added each year. Incidence rates are estimated using statistics from the U.S. Bureau of the Census. The SEER registries routinely collect data on patient demographics, primary tumor site, morphology, stage at diagnosis, first course of treatment, and follow-up for survival.

The **National Registry of Myocardial Infarction (NRMI)** provides information on the current treatment rates at hospitals across the country for patients discharged following myocardial infarction. It is sponsored by Genentech, Inc. More than 1,500 hospitals of all types and from all regions are involved in the registry, and information is collected for more than 5 percent of the total hospitalized acute myocardial infarction (AMI) patients in the United States. NRMI allows hospitals to compare their own treatment rates to this national data set. Since 1990, NRMI has collected data on more than 1.7 million AMI patients.

The **United States Renal Data System (USRDS)** is a national data system that collects, analyzes, and distributes information about the incidence, prevalence, treatment, morbidity, and mortality associated with end-stage renal disease (ESRD). The USRDS is funded directly by the National Institute of Diabetes and Digestive and Kidney Diseases in conjunction with the Centers for Medicare and Medicaid Services. Data are obtained on ESRD patients whose treatment is funded by Medicare, which covers about 93 percent of all treated ESRD patients. Currently, data are available for 581,000 patients treated between 1977 and 1995.

METHODS OF THE SYSTEMATIC LITERATURE REVIEW AND SYNTHESIS

The Committee's literature review updates and broadens the scope of a number of extensive reviews of research measuring the effects of health insurance status on health-related outcomes. Notable prior contributions include *Does Health Insurance Make a Difference,* a background paper prepared by the Congressional

Office of Technology Assessment (OTA, 1992); *Falling Through the Safety Net: Insurance Status and Access to Health Care* (Weissman and Epstein, 1994); "Monitoring the Consequences of Uninsurance: A Review of the Methodologies" (Brown et al., 1998); and *No Health Insurance? It's Enough to Make You Sick* (American College of Physicians–American Society of Internal Medicine, 1999).

To these earlier reviews, the Committee contributes the development and application of explicit criteria used to identify and select studies for inclusion and to assess their methodological strength. This section describes the selection criteria, the evaluation of research quality, and how the individual study findings are presented in Chapter 3.

Identification of Studies and Inclusion Criteria

The systematic literature review includes clinical and health services research and population surveys that are structured to examine the independent effect of health insurance on some health-related outcome. It includes studies with the following dependent variables or outcomes:

- General health status (self-reported or medically evaluated)
- Disease-specific clinical indicators (e.g., blood pressure) and stage of disease at diagnosis or treatment
- Mortality (e.g., in-hospital; longer-term survival rates)
- Functional status, limitations, disability
- Use of services for specific conditions that are associated with improved health outcomes (e.g., periodic dilated eye exams for diabetics)
- Screening and other secondary preventive services
- Use of appropriate procedures (e.g., diagnostic and treatment services after acute myocardial infarction)
- Adverse events due to medical mismanagement
- Hospital admissions for preventable conditions

The Committee excluded those studies that measured only basic access to care (e.g., number of physician visits per year, presence of a regular source of care, difficulty reported in obtaining care when needed) because the relationship between health insurance and access is well established. This literature is discussed earlier in this chapter and in the Committee's first report, *Coverage Matters* (IOM, 2001a).

All studies selected for systematic review include uninsured subjects. Some excluded studies, for example, were limited to comparisons of health-related outcomes among types of insurance coverage (e.g., fee-for-service or indemnity coverage versus health maintenance organization or managed care) and included no information on uninsured patients. The following three categories are the most common classification of insurance status groups for the purposes of the Committee's analysis:

1. privately insured (employment-based or individually purchased coverage);
2. publicly insured (Medicaid, State Children's Health Insurance Program, or Medicare for disabled or end-stage renal disease beneficiaries); and
3. uninsured.

Studies that combine publicly insured and uninsured persons within a single category are included in the literature review because they may offer some insight into the factors that affect health-related outcomes, even though they do not yield results specific to uninsured adults and thus are of limited value in measuring the effects of uninsurance as such. Likewise, studies of health services utilization that report combined results for publicly and privately insured adults are included. Reporting findings for a single category of publicly and privately insured adults also presents a problem for interpretation because these insured groups differ in their health status, with publicly insured adults tending to have worse-than-average health status and privately insured adults better-than-average health status. This difference is rarely adequately controlled for analytically.

The literature review focuses on outcomes for U.S. adults between 18 and 65. This review excludes perinatal and pediatric studies (as noted earlier, these will be reviewed in the next report of the Committee) and studies that are limited to the population over age 65, virtually all of whom have at least medical and hospital insurance, primarily through the Medicare program. To the extent that the research is discussed by disease category (e.g., diabetes care and outcomes), some studies may include children. These studies may be considered in the next Committee report as well.

Almost all of the studies reviewed share a conventional and imprecise definition of health insurance as meaning general medical and hospital coverage. A few of the studies that examine preventive or mental health services assess health-related outcomes as a function of a specific insurance benefit package. These exceptions are noted in the discussion in Chapter 3. Studies that address dental services have been excluded from the review because coverage for dental services is minimal or missing from most basic health insurance plans for adults (KPMG, 1998). Furthermore, studies of dental care and outcomes tend to identify coverage for dental services specifically. Likewise, studies that exclusively consider institutional, long-term, or custodial care as a function of insurance coverage were excluded because these services are not usually included in health insurance benefit packages. Studies of rehabilitation services were included.

The Committee applied its selection criteria to studies identified in PubMed searches conducted between March and June 2001 and updated monthly thereafter through November 2001.[11] Studies cited in the published literature surveys

---

[11]The electronic search included publication dates back to 1965; however, most citations were for studies published after 1985. The search terms included "insurance status," "insurance, longitudinal," "insurance, cohort," "uninsured, longitudinal," "uninsured, cohort," "payer status," "payer source," "medically indigent," and "uncompensated care."

noted earlier in this chapter were also included if they met the criteria set out above. In addition, unpublished studies of which the Committee became aware through experts were included if they met the criteria listed above. A total of 131 primary research studies were reviewed and rated.[12] This primary research bibliography is included in Appendix B.

Evaluation of Research Quality

The goal of the Committee's literature review is to evaluate the nature and quality of the evidence *in the aggregate* for particular kinds of health-related outcomes, rather than to judge the results of specific research studies. Thus, individual studies were evaluated in light of the information that they could contribute to the body of evidence on health insurance effects. To carry out that evaluation, two reviewers rated each study in the research bibliography (see Appendix B). Box 2-5 presents the methodological review criteria. One reviewer was a member of the Subcommittee on Health Outcomes for the Uninsured and the other was an Institute of Medicine staff member or consultant with training complementary to that of the first reviewer. Studies that were judged to be of poor quality by both reviewers were not used in formulating the Committee's findings. If studies were judged to be of fair or good methodological quality by one reviewer and poor by the other, they were submitted to a third reviewer (a Subcommittee or Committee member). Quantitative results are presented in Chapters 3 and 4 only for studies that received a fair or good evaluation from two reviewers.

Presentation of Committee Findings

Chapter 3 presents the Committee's findings based on the literature review, with the evaluation of studies organized into categories that reflect either specific diseases or type of service such as preventive and screening services or hospital care. The categories reflect practical considerations, including ease of presentation and summary of results. Findings regarding specific health conditions are more easily understood within the context of similar clinical research and can be related to larger populations at risk. Service-based categories permit synthesis of findings across studies with consistent outcome measures. This may be especially useful because health insurance coverage rules are often structured by service categories (e.g., preventive and screening services may be excluded or covered without any cost sharing to promote their use) but may also specify exclusions based on condition (e.g., mental illness).

---

[12]Separate articles using the same sample and analytic design, as noted in Appendix B, are counted as a single study here.

BOX 2.5
Study Methodology Review Criteria

The methodological quality of each study was rated on a three-point scale: Good = 3, Fair = 2, or Poor = 1. These ratings were based on the following considerations:

• The validity and relevance of the outcome measure (e.g., whether the study provides information on a result that is of interest). For example, if a process-of-care or preventive service measure was the focus of the study (the dependent variable), does an evidence base link it to a health outcome? If a health outcome is the dependent variable, is reporting of that outcome unbiased and reliable?

• Whether the health insurance status categories are well defined and consistently reported. For example, is health insurance status directly measured?

• The adequacy of adjustments to minimize biases introduced by covariates of health insurance status. At a minimum, studies should adjust or control for age, sex, and race–ethnicity. It should be noted, however, that by controlling for social and demographic covariates (e.g., race–ethnicity), cumulative effects or interactions between such factors and health insurance status may be missed in the analysis. Ideally, variables measuring income or educational attainment, health status, and site of care (for a process or quality-of-care outcome measure) should be included. In ranking a study's quality, reviewers determined which of these likely covariates were most important, given the specific outcome being measured.

• The study design, including consideration of the sample size, response rate, amount of missing data, representativeness of the study population, and consideration given to potential selection biases.

In developing its summary findings, the Committee considered the volume of evidence within a given category in terms of the number and representativeness of studies and the degree of consistency among studies. The Committee gave greater weight to longitudinal than to cross-sectional studies and, among cross-sectional studies, placed more importance on those that measured and appropriately considered key covariates. Regardless of the Committee's evaluation of methodological quality, however, all studies with results inconsistent with the Committee's summary findings are discussed in Chapter 3 and included in Appendix B.

NOTES

BOX 3.1
Summary of Findings

- The Committee finds a consistent and statistically significant relationship between health insurance coverage and health outcomes for adults. Coverage is associated with having a regular source of care, which promotes continuity of care, and with greater use of appropriate health services. These factors, in turn, improve the likelihood of disease screening and early detection, the management of chronic illness, and the treatment of acute conditions such as traumatic injury and heart attacks. The ultimate result is improved health outcomes.

- The most compelling evidence for the difference that health insurance can make in health outcomes is in chronic disease care and in prevention and screening. Studies of acutely ill or injured patients and of the general mortality experience of insured and uninsured populations also provide evidence for concluding that health outcomes are better for privately insured than for uninsured adults.

- Health insurance is most likely to improve health outcomes if the coverage is continuous and enrollees have access to high-quality providers and sites of care with adequate facilities and services. While Medicaid has been found to improve access to and use of services, it is not always associated with better health outcomes. The Committee concludes that this lesser effectiveness of Medicaid with respect to health outcomes is in part due to the intermittent nature of the coverage it provides.

3

Effects of Health Insurance on Health

This chapter presents the Committee's review of studies that address the impact of health insurance on various health-related outcomes. It examines research on the relationship between health insurance (or lack of insurance), use of medical care and health outcomes for specific conditions and types of services, and with overall health status and mortality. There is a consistent, positive relationship between health insurance coverage and health-related outcomes across a body of studies that use a variety of data sources and different analytic approaches. The best evidence suggests that health insurance is associated with more appropriate use of health care services and better health outcomes for adults.

The discussion of the research in this chapter is organized within sections that encompass virtually all of the research literature on health outcomes and insurance status that the Committee identified. The chapter sections include the following:

- Primary prevention and screening services
- Cancer care and outcomes
- Chronic disease management, with specific discussions of diabetes, hypertension, end-stage renal disease (ESRD), HIV disease, and mental illness
- Hospital-based care (emergency services, traumatic injury, cardiovascular disease)
- Overall mortality and general measures of health status

The Committee consolidated study results within categories that reflect both diseases and services because these frameworks helped in summarizing the individual studies and subsumed similar research structures and outcome measures. Older studies and those of lesser relevance or quality are not discussed within this chapter devoted to presenting study results and reaching Committee findings. However, all of the studies reviewed are described briefly in Appendix B.

The studies presented in some detail in this chapter are those that the Committee judged to be both methodologically sound and the most informative regarding health insurance effects on health-related outcomes.[1] Most studies report a positive relationship between health insurance coverage and measured outcomes. However, all studies with negative results that are contrary to the Committee's findings are presented and discussed in this chapter. Appendix B includes summaries of the complete set of studies that the Committee reviewed.

In the pages that follow, the Committee's findings introduce each of the five major sections listed above and also some of the subsections under chronic disease and hospital-based care. All of the Committee's specific findings are also presented together in Box 3.12 in the concluding section of this chapter. These findings are the basis for the Committee's overall conclusions in Chapter 4.

PRIMARY PREVENTION AND SCREENING SERVICES

Finding: Uninsured adults are less likely than adults with any kind of health coverage to receive preventive and screening services and less likely to receive these services on a timely basis. Health insurance that provides more extensive coverage of preventive and screening services is likely to result in greater and more appropriate use of these services.

Finding: Health insurance may reduce racial and ethnic disparities in the receipt of preventive and screening services.

These findings have important implications for health outcomes, as can be seen in the later sections on cancer and chronic diseases. For prevention and screening services, health insurance facilitates both the receipt of services and a continuing care relationship or regular source of care, which also increases the likelihood of receiving appropriate care.

Insurance benefits are less likely to include preventive and screening services (Box 3.2) than they are physician visits for acute care or diagnostic tests for symptomatic conditions. However, over time, coverage of preventive and screen-

---

[1]Chapter 2 discusses the features of observational (nonexperimental) studies that are necessary for methodological soundness. All quantified study results that are presented in this chapter and in Chapter 4 are significant at least at the 95 percent confidence interval. If results do not meet this level of statistical significance, the confidence interval is reported. See "confidence interval" in Appendix C for further discussion.

BOX 3.2
Screening Services

The U.S. Preventive Services Task Force (USPSTF) recommends screening for the following conditions in the general adult population under age 65: cervical cancer (above age 18), breast and colorectal cancer (above age 50), hypertension (all ages), and high cholesterol (men over 35 and women over 45) (USPSTF, 1996; Coffield et al., 2001). These evidence-based standards are updated periodically to reflect both the extent of clinically preventable disease and the cost-effectiveness of the services.

These standards are the basis for comparing the receipt of appropriate preventive services by insured and uninsured adults in the studies whose results are discussed in this chapter. They include the following:

• Papanicolaou (Pap) tests (for cervical cancer) in women 18 and older at least every three years,
• Clinical breast exam and mammography in women aged 50 to 69 at least every two years,
• Fecal occult blood test (for colorectal cancer) at least every two years for persons ages 50 to 64,
• Sigmoidoscopy (for colorectal cancer) at least every five years for persons ages 50 to 64,*
• Blood pressure check annually (for hypertension) for all adults, and
• Cholesterol test at least every five years for men over 35 and women over 45.

Studies of utilization of preventive and screening services are usually based on population surveys and self-reporting rather than on clinical or billing records.

---

*Frequency recommended by American Gastroenterological Association (Winawer et al., 1997).

ing services has been increasing. In 1998, about three-quarters of adults with employment-based health insurance had a benefit package that included adult physical examinations; two years later in 2000, the proportion had risen to 90 percent (KPMG, 1998; Kaiser Family Foundation/HRET, 2000). Yet even if health insurance benefit packages do not cover preventive or screening services, those with health insurance are more likely to receive these recommended services because they are more likely to have a regular source of care, and having a regular source of care is independently associated with receiving recommended services (Bush and Langer, 1998; Gordon et al., 1998; Mandelblatt et al., 1999; Zambrana et al., 1999; Cummings et al., 2000; Hsia et al., 2000; Breen et al., 2001). The effect of having health insurance is more evident for relatively costly services, such as mammograms, than for less costly services, such as a clinical breast exam (CBE) or Pap test (Zambrana et al., 1999; Cummings et al., 2000; O'Malley et al., 2001).

According to several large population surveys conducted within the past decade, adults without health insurance are less likely to receive recommended preventive and screening services and are less likely to receive them at the frequencies recommended by the United States Preventive Services Task Force than are insured adults.[2] The 1992 National Health Interview Survey (NHIS) documented receipt of mammography, CBE, Pap test, fecal occult blood test (FOBT), sigmoidoscopy, and digital rectal exam by adults under 65 (Potosky et al., 1998). Those with no health insurance had significantly lower screening rates compared to those with private coverage *and* compared to those with Medicaid for every service except sigmoidoscopy. The odds ratios (ORs) for receiving a screening service if uninsured compared with having private health insurance ranged from 0.27 for mammography to 0.43 for Pap test.[3]

The 1998 NHIS found that, although rates of screening at appropriate intervals had increased generally over the preceding decade, they remained substantially lower for uninsured adults than for those with any kind of health insurance (Breen et al., 2001).[4] In a multivariable analysis that adjusted for age, race, education, and a regular source of care, uninsured adults were significantly less likely than those with any kind of coverage to receive a Pap test, mammography, and colorectal screening (FOBT or sigmoidoscopy) (ORs ranged from 0.37 to 0.5) (Breen et al., 2001). The study reported a strong relationship between having a regular source of care and timely receipt of these screening services in addition to the relationship between health insurance and screening.

Studies using other national samples report results consistent with those of the NHIS. A study of more than 31,000 women between ages 50 and 64 who responded to telephone surveys conducted between 1994 and 1997 about their receipt of mammograms, Pap smears, and colorectal cancer screening (either FOBT or sigmoidoscopy) found that uninsured women were significantly less likely to

---

[2]Earlier studies based on the 1986 Access to Care Survey and the 1982 NHIS had findings consistent with those of the more recent nationally representative sample surveys regarding receipt of preventive and screening services by those without health insurance (Hayward et al., 1988; Woolhandler and Himmelstein, 1988).

[3]Enrollees in private managed care plans is the reference group; however, fee-for-service enrollees did not have significantly different screening rates from those of managed care enrollees. The odds ratio is the relative odds of having an outcome in the uninsured and insured groups. For example, if the odds of receiving a Pap test are 2:1 in a group of uninsured women (i.e., two of every three women or 67 percent receive the test) and the odds are 4:1 in a group of women with insurance (i.e., four of every five women, or 80 percent, receive the test), the odds ratio of uninsured compared to insured women is 0.5 (2:1/4:1). The OR is not a good estimate of the relative risk (the probability of been screened in the uninsured group divided by the probability of being screened in the insured group) because screening is not a rare event. Throughout this report the results of particular studies, if reported as odds ratios or as relative risks, will be presented as the ratio of the uninsured to the insured rates (in this example, as an OR of 0.5).

[4]Comparing results presented in Potosky et al., 1998, and Breen et al., 2001, the gap in screening rates between insured and uninsured adults decreased between 1992 and 1998.

have received these tests than were women with private prepaid plan insurance (ORs ranging from 0.30 to 0.50) (Hsia et al., 2000). This study also found a strong relationship between having a regular source of care and receipt of screening services. Health insurance was an independently significant predictor. Another study based on several years of the Behavioral Risk Factor Surveillance System (BRFSS) for older adults (55 through 64) found that uninsured men and women were much less likely than their insured counterparts to receive cancer or heart disease screening tests and also much less likely to have a regular source of care (Powell-Griner et al., 1999; see Table 4.1).

Disparities Among Population Groups

A review of the literature on the interaction of race, ethnicity, and socioeconomic status (SES) with health insurance, concluded that health insurance makes a positive contribution to the likelihood of receiving appropriate screening services, although racial and ethnic disparities persist independent of health insurance (Haas and Adler, 2001). Studies of the use of preventive services by particular ethnic groups, such as Hispanics and African Americans, find that health insurance is associated with increased receipt of preventive services and increased likelihood of having a regular source of care, which improves one's chances of receiving appropriate preventive services (Solis et al., 1990; Mandelblatt et al., 1999; Zambrana et al., 1999; Wagner and Guendelman, 2000; Breen et al., 2001; O'Malley et al., 2001).

Breen and colleagues (2001) modeled the expected increase in screening rates for different ethnic groups if they were to gain health insurance coverage and a regular source of care. This "what-if" model suggests that those groups for whom screening rates are particularly low (e.g., receipt of mammography by Hispanic women, colorectal screening of African-American men) would make the largest gains (an 11 percentage-point increase in mammography rates for Hispanic women [to 77 percent] and a 5 percentage-point increase in colorectal screening for African-American men [to 31 percent] (Breen et al., 2001).

Extensiveness of Insurance Benefits

The type of health insurance and the continuity of coverage have also been found to affect receipt of appropriate preventive and screening services. Faulkner and Schauffler (1997) examined receipt of physical examinations, blood pressure screening, lipid screening for detection of cardiovascular disease, Pap test, CBE, and mammography and identified a positive and statistically significant "dose–response" relationship between the extent of coverage for preventive services (e.g., whether all such services, most, some, or none were covered by health insurance). Insurance coverage for preventive care increased men's receipt of preventive services more than it did that of women. Men with no coverage for preventive services were much less likely than men with complete coverage for such services to receive them (ORs for receipt of specific services ranged from 0.36 to 0.56). Women with no preventive services coverage also received fewer of these services than did women with full coverage for them (ORs for specific services ranged from 0.5 to 0.83) (Faulkner and Schauffler, 1997).

Ayanian and colleagues (2000) used the 1998 BRFSS data set to analyze the effect of length of time without coverage on receipt of preventive and screening services for adults between ages 18 and 65. Those without coverage for a year or longer were more likely than those uninsured for less than one year to go without appropriate preventive and screening services. For every generally recommended service (mammography, CBE, Pap smear, FOBT, sigmoidoscopy, hypertension screening, and cholesterol screening), the longer-term uninsured were significantly less likely than persons with any form of health insurance to receive these services (Ayanian et al., 2000).

Negative Findings

In the Committee's review, the one study that did not find a positive effect of insurance coverage compared mammography use among clients of various sites of care in Detroit, Michigan: two health department clinics, a health maintenance organization (HMO), and a private hospital (Burack et al., 1993). This study found no significant differences among women according to their health insurance status but did find that patients with more visits annually for any service (seven or more) were more likely to receive mammography. All women in this study had access to a primary care provider and, in the case of uninsured women, to clinics with the mission of serving the uninsured. These factors may explain why uninsured women had mammography rates as high as those of women with insurance.

CANCER CARE AND OUTCOMES

Finding: Uninsured cancer patients generally have poorer outcomes and are more likely to die prematurely than persons with insurance, largely because of delayed diagnosis. This finding is supported by population-based studies of breast, cervical, colorectal, and prostate cancer and melanoma.

The studies analyzing health-related outcomes for cancer patients provide some of the most compelling evidence for the effect of health insurance status on health outcomes (Box 3.3). This evidence comes from research based on area or statewide cancer registries, which provide large numbers of observations and reflect almost all cases occurring in a geographic region. Multivariable data analysis is used to determine the independent effects of health insurance, by controlling for demographic, SES, and clinical differences among study subjects.

In addition to receiving fewer cancer screening services, uninsured adults are at greater risk of late-stage, often fatal cancer. Early diagnosis frequently improves

> **BOX 3.3**
> **Cancer**
>
> • Cancers of all kinds have an overall incidence nationally of 400 cases per 100,000 people each year. More than 8.9 million Americans alive today have a history of cancer. Cancers account for approximately 550,000 deaths each year in the United States and are the second leading cause of death (NCHS, 2001; NCI-SEER, 2001).*
> • Breast cancer is by far the most prevalent cancer among American women, and the second most common cause of cancer-related deaths, more than 40,000 each year, among women. During the 1990s, almost 2 million women were diagnosed with breast cancer. Eighty percent of breast cancers occur among women over 50. An estimated 30 percent of breast cancer deaths, about 13,000 annually, could be prevented if women age 50 and older received regular mammograms (CDC, 1999b).
> • Colorectal cancer is the second leading cause (after lung cancer) of cancer-related deaths for the U.S. population overall, accounting for 57,000 deaths annually.
> • Prostate cancer accounts for almost a third of all cancer cases in men and is the second leading cause of cancer-related deaths in men, accounting for 31,500 deaths annually.
> • Cancer survival is related largely to stage of the disease at the time it is diagnosed.
> • Stage of disease at diagnosis and mortality rates are the predominant outcome measures in studies that examine the effects of health insurance status on cancer care and outcomes.
>
> _____
>
> *Actual for 1999 and projected for 2001.

the chances of surviving cancer. Generally, in studies examining the stage at which cancer is diagnosed, those with private health insurance have the best outcomes and those with no insurance have the worst (i.e., the highest proportion of late-stage diagnoses), with intermediate outcomes for Medicaid enrollees. In some studies however, the outcomes for Medicaid enrollees are comparable to those for uninsured cancer patients (Roetzheim et al., 1999). Both because of an assumption of similarity in SES between uninsured and Medicaid patients and because of small numbers of observations in the separate categories, some studies report combined results for Medicaid and uninsured patients and compare these findings with those for privately insured patients (e.g., Lee-Feldstein et al., 2000).

In studies assessing the outcomes for adults with cancer—stage of disease at diagnosis and mortality—Medicaid enrollees often do no better, and sometimes do worse, than uninsured patients. This similarity in experience between patients enrolled in Medicaid and those without any coverage may reflect the fact that uninsured persons in poor health, once they seek care, may become enrolled in

Medicaid as a result of their frequent interactions with the health care system (Davidoff et al., 2001; see Box 2.1). Also, Medicaid enrollees tend to have discontinuous coverage and thus may have had less regular access to screening services. Consequently, persons with Medicaid at the time of a cancer diagnosis may have been without coverage for some prior period (Carrasquillo et al., 1998; IOM, 2001a; Perkins et al., 2001). For example, one study of women under 65 with Medi-Cal coverage (California's Medicaid and indigent care program) who were diagnosed with breast cancer found that, among those who had been uninsured during the year prior to their diagnosis (18 percent of all Medi-Cal enrollees), late-stage diagnosis was much more likely than among those who had been continuously enrolled for the previous 12 months (ORs of 3.9 for those who had been uninsured and 1.4 for those continuously covered by Medi-Cal, compared with all other women ages 30–64 diagnosed with breast cancer) (Perkins et al., 2001).

With this general background on the nature of the research examining health insurance status effects, the remainder of this section discusses study results for five specific cancers.

Breast Cancer

Uninsured women and women with Medicaid are more likely to receive a breast cancer diagnosis at a late stage of disease (regional or distant) and have a 30–50 percent greater risk of dying than women with private coverage, as shown in studies based on three different state or regional cancer registries (Ayanian et al., 1993; Roetzheim et al., 1999, 2000; Lee-Feldstein et al., 2000).

In a study using the New Jersey Cancer Registry, Ayanian and colleagues (1993) identified 4,675 women 35 to 65 years of age diagnosed with breast cancer and assessed their stage of disease at diagnosis and their survival rates 4.5 to 7 years after diagnosis. The authors found that uninsured women were significantly more likely than privately insured women to be diagnosed with regional or late-stage cancer, as were patients with Medicaid. After controlling for stage of disease at diagnosis and other factors, uninsured women had an adjusted risk of death 49 percent higher than that of privately insured women, and women with Medicaid had a 40 percent higher risk of death than those who were privately insured.

Using a regional cancer registry and Census data for 1987 through 1993, Lee-Feldstein and colleagues (2000) examined the stage of disease at diagnosis, treatment, and survival experience of about 1,800 northern California women under the age of 65 diagnosed with breast cancer. They found that women who were uninsured and publicly insured (primarily Medicaid), taken together, were twice as likely as privately insured women with indemnity coverage to be diagnosed at a late stage of disease. Over a four- to ten-year follow-up, uninsured and publicly insured women had higher risks of death from both breast cancer (42 percent higher) and all causes (46 percent higher) than did privately insured women with indemnity coverage. The likelihood of receiving breast-conserving surgery did not differ between these two groups.

In a review of approximately 9,800 Florida residents diagnosed with breast cancer in 1994, Roetzheim and colleagues calculated that, after controlling for age, education, income, marital status, race, and comorbidity, women without insurance were more likely to be diagnosed with late-stage disease than women with private indemnity coverage (OR = 1.43) (Roetzheim et al., 1999). Women with Medicaid had an even greater likelihood of late-stage diagnosis compared with privately insured women (OR = 1.87). In a subsequent analysis of mortality using the same registry data, the authors estimated that the relative risk (RR) of dying was 31 percent higher for uninsured women and 58 percent higher for women with Medicaid over a three to four-year follow-up period (Roetzheim et al, 2000a). Further analysis suggested that stage of disease at diagnosis and, to a lesser extent, treatment modality appeared to account for the differences in survival by insurance status. Finally, uninsured women were less likely than women with private coverage to receive breast-conserving surgery when stage at diagnosis, comorbidities, and other personal characteristics were taken into account (OR = 0.70) (Roetzheim et al., 2000a).

Cervical Cancer

Uninsured women are more likely to receive a late-stage diagnosis for invasive cervical cancer than are privately insured women. Ferrante and colleagues (2000) analyzed 852 cases of invasive cervical cancer reported in the Florida tumor registry for 1994 to determine factors associated with late-stage diagnosis. In bivariate analysis, being uninsured was associated with an increased likelihood of late-stage diagnosis (OR = 1.6). In a multivariable analysis that adjusted for age, education, income, marital status, race, comorbidities, and smoking, uninsured women were more likely to present with a late-stage cancer compared to women with private indemnity coverage, although this finding was not statistically significant (OR = 1.49, confidence interval [CI]: 0.88–2.50). The outcome for Medicaid enrollees was similar to that of privately insured women in both bivariate and multivariable analysis (Ferrante et al., 2000).

Colorectal Cancer

Uninsured patients with colorectal cancer have a greater risk of dying than do patients with private indemnity insurance, even after adjusting for differences in the stage at which the cancer is diagnosed and the treatment modality. Using the Florida cancer registry for 1994, Roetzheim and colleagues (1999) analyzed the relative likelihood of late-stage diagnosis by insurance status for more than 8,000 cases of colorectal cancer. In a multivariable analysis adjusting for sociodemographic characteristics, smoking status, and comorbidities, uninsured patients were more likely to be diagnosed with late-stage colorectal cancer than were patients with private indemnity coverage (OR = 1.67). Medicaid enrollees had a statistically insignificant greater likelihood of late-stage disease compared to patients with indemnity coverage (OR = 1.44, CI: 0.92–2.25).

A subsequent analysis of largely the same data set (9,500 cases) that adjusted for sociodemographic factors and comorbidities but not for smoking estimated the adjusted mortality risk for uninsured patients with colorectal cancer to be 64 percent greater over a three- to four-year follow-up period than that for patients covered by private indemnity plans (Roetzheim et al., 2000b).[5] Even after adjusting for stage of disease at diagnosis, the risk of death for uninsured patients was 50 percent higher than that for the privately insured, and after further adjustment for treatment modality, the risk for uninsured patients was 40 percent higher (Roetzheim et al., 2000b).

Prostate Cancer

In addition to delayed diagnosis and greater risk of death, uninsured prostate cancer patients have been found to experience a decrease in health-related quality of life after their diagnosis and during treatment, unlike publicly and privately insured patients. A study of about 8,700 cases of newly diagnosed prostate cancer reported to the Florida cancer registry in 1994 found that uninsured men were more likely to be diagnosed at a late stage of the disease than were men with private indemnity insurance (OR = 1.47) (Roetzheim et al., 1999). A study of 860 men in 26 medical practices with newly diagnosed prostate cancer evaluated their health-related quality of life (HRQOL) at three- to six-month intervals over a two-year period (Penson et al., 2001). Although uninsured men diagnosed with prostate cancer did not have a lower HRQOL at diagnosis, their HRQOL decreased over the course of their disease and treatment, in contrast to that of HMO and Medicare patients. The authors suggest that "patients undergoing aggressive treatment, which can itself have deleterious effects on quality of life, are exposed to further hardships when they do not have comprehensive health insurance upon which to support their care" (Penson et al., 2001, p. 357).

Melanoma

Uninsured patients, as well as Medicaid patients have been found to be more likely to be diagnosed with late-stage melanoma than are privately insured patients. Among 1,500 patients diagnosed with melanoma, uninsured patients were more likely to have late-stage (regional or distant) disease than those with private indemnity coverage (OR = 2.6) (Roetzheim et al., 1999). The small number of Medicaid patients with melanoma (13) included in this study also had a much greater chance of being diagnosed with late-stage cancer.

---

[5]Smoking has been associated with an increased risk of colorectal cancer (Chao et al., 2000).

> ### BOX 3.4
> ### Chronic Conditions
>
> • Chronic conditions are the leading causes of death, disability, and illness in the United States, accounting for one-third of the potential life years lost before age 65 (CDC, 2000a). Almost 100 million Americans have chronic conditions. The aging of the population will increase the prevalence of such health impairments over time (NAAS, 1999).
> • Among middle-aged adults, hypertension, arthritis, and orthopedic impairments are the most common chronic health conditions (NAAS, 1999).
> • Chronic conditions such as hypertension, diabetes, and arthritis are more prevalent among lower-income adults and members of racial and ethnic minorities, who report worse functioning with these conditions than do higher-income or white adults (Kington and Smith, 1997; NAAS, 1999).
> • Studies of the effects of health insurance on chronic disease care and outcomes frequently examine provider visits at appropriate intervals, receipt of specific diagnostic or treatment services (e.g., measurement of blood pressure and antihypertensive medication for someone diagnosed with high blood pressure), and specific clinical outcomes (e.g., blood pressure control over time).

CHRONIC DISEASE CARE AND OUTCOMES

Finding: Uninsured people with chronic diseases are less likely to receive appropriate care to manage their health conditions than are those who have health insurance. For the five disease conditions that the Committee examined (diabetes, cardiovascular disease, end-stage renal disease, HIV infection, and mental illness), uninsured patients have worse clinical outcomes than insured patients.

Effective management of chronic conditions such as diabetes, hypertension, HIV, and depression (Box 3.4) includes not only periodic services and care from health care professionals but also the active involvement of patients in modifying their behavior, monitoring their condition, and participating in treatment regimens (Wagner et al., 1996; Davis et al., 2000). Identifying chronic conditions early and providing appropriate health care on an ongoing and coordinated basis are health care system goals that have been developed over several decades and have been continuously refined as evidence for cost-effective interventions and practices has accumulated. Maintaining an ongoing relationship with a specific provider who keeps records, manages care, and is available for consultation between visits is a key to high-quality health care, particularly for those with chronic illnesses (O'Connor et al., 1998; IOM, 2001b).

For persons with a chronic illness, health insurance may be most important in that it enhances the opportunities to acquire a regular source of care. If someone has coverage through a private or public managed care plan, a relationship with a primary care provider may be built into the insurance. Indemnity or fee-for-service (FFS) insurance coverage also improves the chances of having a regular source of care because having the resources to pay for services is often a prerequisite to being seen in a medical practice. Uninsured adults are much less likely to have a regular source of care and are more likely to identify an emergency department as their regular source of care than are adults with any form of coverage (Weinick et al., 1997; Cunningham and Whitmore, 1998; Zuvekas and Weinick, 1999; Haley and Zuckerman, 2000). Loss of coverage also interrupts patterns of use of health care and results in delays in seeking needed care (Burstin et al., 1998; Kasper et al., 2000; Hoffman et al., 2001). For uninsured adults under age 65, 19 percent with heart disease and 14 percent with hypertension lack a usual source of care, compared to 8 and 4 percent, respectively, of their insured counterparts (Fish-Parcham, 2001). For uninsured patients without a regular source of care or those who identify an emergency department as their usual source, obtaining care that is consistent with recognized standards for effective disease management is a daunting challenge.

Providers with a commitment to serving uninsured clients, such as local public health and hospital clinics and federally funded community health centers, have sometimes instituted special interventions and programs for the chronically ill to promote continuity of care and disease management. These innovations are critically important to the identified, chronically ill patients who routinely receive care at such clinics and centers. The efforts of these providers, however, are limited in scale by funding and service capacity relative to the high need for care within their service areas (Baker et al., 1998; Chin et al., 2000; Piette, 2000; Philis-Tsimikas and Walker, 2001). As demonstrated in the following review of studies examining the care and outcomes for patients with specific chronic conditions, those who do not have health insurance coverage of any kind fare measurably worse than their insured counterparts.

Cardiovascular Disease

Finding: Uninsured adults with hypertension or high cholesterol have diminished access to care, are less likely to be screened, are less likely to take prescription medication if diagnosed, and experience worse health outcomes.

Across the spectrum of services and the course of development of cardiovascular disease (Box 3.5), uninsured adults receive fewer services and experience worse health. They are less likely to receive screening for hypertension and high cholesterol and to have frequent monitoring of blood pressure once they develop hypertension. Uninsured adults are less likely to stay on drug therapy for hypertension both because they lack a regular provider and because they do not have

> **BOX 3.5**
> **Cardiovascular Disease**
>
> • "Cardiovascular disease" encompasses a variety of diseases and condi-
> tions that affect the heart and blood vessels, including hypertension (high blood
> pressure), heart disease, and stroke.
> • One-quarter of all Americans have cardiovascular disease, and 960,000 die
> from it each year, more than 40 percent of all deaths in the United States (CDC,
> 2001b).
> • Hypertension is a major risk factor for heart disease and stroke, two of the
> leading causes of death, and affects more than 50 million Americans (Burt et al.,
> 1995).
> • Of adults ages 45 to 55, 18 percent have hypertension, with the prevalence
> of the condition rising to 29 percent of all persons between ages 55 and 65 (Kilker,
> 2000). In the latter age group, African Americans have twice the prevalence of
> hypertension (52 percent) as do whites (26 percent).
> • High cholesterol blood levels also contribute to cardiovascular disease. A
> third of American adults need either dietary modification or lipid-lowering medica-
> tion for high blood cholesterol.
> • Hypertension screening (blood pressure measurement) is recommended
> for all adults annually (USPSTF, 1996). Cholesterol screening is recommended
> for all men over 35 and women over 45 at least once every five years (USPSTF,
> 1996).
> • Studies examining care and outcomes for cardiovascular disease measure
> the adequacy of blood pressure control, frequency of visits, and mortality.

insurance coverage. Loss of insurance coverage has been demonstrated to disrupt therapeutic relationships and worsen control of blood pressure.

Uninsured adults are less likely to receive routine screening services for cardiovascular disease. A nationwide household survey in 1997 found that adults who had been without health insurance for one year or longer were less likely than insured adults to have received recommended hypertension screening within the previous two years (80 percent compared with 94 percent) or cholesterol screening (60 percent compared with 82 percent) (Ayanian et al., 2000). Adults who were uninsured for less than one year received these screening services at rates intermediate between those for long-term uninsured and insured adults.

Health insurance coverage is associated with better blood pressure control for lower-income persons with hypertension, according to two studies, one prospective and experimental and the other a longitudinal analysis of a cohort of patients that either lost or maintained Medicaid coverage. The prospective study, the RAND Health Insurance Experiment, found that for patients with diagnosed hypertension, patients in the plan without any cost sharing had significantly lower blood pressure than those in health plans with any form of cost sharing (an overall difference of 1.9 mm Hg) (Keeler et al., 1985). A much greater effect of cost sharing on average blood pressure was found for low-income patients than for high-income patients (3.5 mm Hg. versus 1.1 mm Hg.). Patients in the plan without cost sharing also had greater compliance with drug and behavioral therapies. These differences were attributed to more frequent contact with health providers in the free care plan (Keeler et al., 1985).[6]

In the longitudinal analysis, Lurie and colleagues (1984, 1986) followed a cohort of patients at a university ambulatory care clinic for one year after some lost their Medi-Cal coverage consequent to a state policy change. At six months after loss of coverage and again at one year, hypertensive patients who lost coverage had significantly worse blood pressure than did those who remained covered by Medi-Cal, with an average increase in diastolic blood pressure of 6 mm Hg compared with a decrease in the insured control group of 3 mm Hg after a full year (Lurie et al., 1984, 1986). The percentage of patients with diastolic blood pressure greater than 100 mm Hg increased in the group that lost coverage from 3 percent at baseline to 31 percent at six months, and then declined to 19 percent at one year, while the proportion with diastolic blood pressure > 100 mm Hg in the continuously covered control group did not change significantly over the year (Lurie et al., 1986).

Deficits in the care of uninsured persons with hypertension place them at risk of complications and deterioration in their condition. The 1987 National Medical Expenditures Survey afforded an in-depth examination of the use of antihypertensive medications by health insurance status. Uninsured persons younger than 65 who had hypertension were less likely than either those with private insurance or Medicaid to have any antihypertensive medication therapy (ORs = 0.62 and 0.44, respectively) (Huttin et al., 2000).[7] An analysis of the third round of the National Health and Nutrition Examination Survey (NHANES), with data on 40,000 respondents for the period 1988–1994, found that 22 percent of uninsured adults under age 65 with diagnosed hypertension had gone for more than one year without a blood pressure check, compared to 10 percent of insured adults with hypertension (Fish-Parcham, 2001). While 75 percent of insured adults under 65 who had ever been diagnosed with high blood pressure and been told to take medication for it were in fact taking blood pressure medication, only 58 percent of

---

[6]This hypertension result was an exception to the overall results for the RAND study, which did not find significant differences in outcomes for most conditions and dimensions of health. These results are discussed further in the General Health Outcomes section later in this chapter.

[7]Notably, this same study found that persons with hypertension who had Medicare coverage only (which does not pay for outpatient prescription drugs) did not have a statistically significant difference in their likelihood of receiving antihypertensive medication than uninsured persons, while those who had Medicare plus Medicaid coverage or Medicare with private supplemental insurance were significantly more likely to have received drug therapy than uninsured persons with hypertension.

their uninsured counterparts who had been advised to take medication were doing so. Among those adults under 65 who had been advised to take cholesterol-lowering medication, 43 percent of those without insurance failed to take such medication, compared to 29 percent among those with health insurance who did not comply with this advice (Fish-Parcham, 2001).

A study by Shea and colleagues (1992a, 1992b) of patients presenting to two New York hospital emergency departments between 1989 and 1991 found that uninsured patients were more likely to have severe, uncontrolled hypertension than were sociodemographically similar patients with any health insurance (OR = 2.2), while patients without a regular source of care had an even greater risk of severe and uncontrolled disease (OR = 4.4). When insurance status, having a regular source of care, and complying with a therapeutic regimen were all included in the analysis, the odds ratio for being uninsured was no longer statistically significant (OR = 1.9, CI: 0.8–4.6). This result is not surprising, given the strong association between having health insurance and having a regular source of care.

Diabetes

> **Finding: Uninsured persons with diabetes are less likely to receive recommended services. Lacking health insurance for longer periods increases the risk of inadequate care for this condition and can lead to uncontrolled blood sugar levels, which, over time, put diabetics at risk for additional chronic disease and disability.**

Despite the demanding and costly care regimen that persons with diabetes face, adults with diabetes are almost as likely to lack health insurance as those without this disease. Of diabetic adults under age 65, 12 percent are uninsured compared with 15 percent of the comparable general population (Harris, 1999). Persons with diabetes who are uninsured are less likely to receive the professionally recommended standard of care than are those who have health insurance (Box 3.6). One result of not receiving appropriate care may be uncontrolled blood sugar levels, which puts diabetics at increased risk of hospitalization for either hyper- or hypoglycemia, in addition to increasing the likelihood of comorbidities and disabilities (Palta et al., 1997).

Based on a 1994 survey, among adults diagnosed with diabetes who did not use insulin, those without health insurance were less likely than those with any kind of coverage to self-monitor blood glucose (OR = 0.5) or, within the past year, to have had their feet examined (OR = 0.4), or a dilated eye exam (OR = 0.5) (Beckles et al., 1998).[8] Persons with diabetes who used insulin and were

---

[8]BRFSS has documented the use of recommended services among insured and uninsured persons with diabetes for two recent years. BRFSS collected information on diabetes management in 1994 in 22 jurisdictions (21 states and the District of Columbia) and in 1998 in 37 jurisdictions, representing 70 percent of the U.S. population (Beckles et al., 1998; Ayanian et al., 2000).

BOX 3.6
Diabetes

- Diabetes mellitus is a prevalent chronic disease that has been increasing in the U.S. population by 5–6 percent each year during the past decade. Approximately 800,000 new cases are diagnosed each year.*
- More than 16 million Americans have diabetes, about one-third of whom have not been diagnosed and are unaware that they have it.
- Diabetes contributes to heart disease, stroke, blindness, hypertension, kidney disease, and amputations and is the seventh leading cause of death.
- Diabetes disproportionately affects minority populations; its prevalence is 10 percent among African Americans, 8 percent among Hispanics, and just over 6 percent among whites. African Americans with diabetes have a significantly higher risk of death than do whites with diabetes (Gu et al., 1998).
- Standards of care for adults with diabetes include receipt of formal diabetes self-management education upon diagnosis, pneumococcal immunization, and the following services at least annually: a glycosylated hemoglobin (blood glucose) measurement, dilated eye examination, foot examination, lipid tests, microalbuminuria screening, and influenza immunization (American Diabetes Association, 2000; USDHHS, 2000).

---

*Unless otherwise noted, statistics cited are from CDC (1999a).

---

uninsured were also less likely than those with health insurance to have had a foot examination (OR = 0.25) or a dilated eye examination (OR = 0.34) (Beckles et al., 1998).

A later analysis, using 1998 data from the same annual survey, found that 25 percent of adults younger than 65 who had diabetes and were uninsured for a year or more had not had a routine checkup within the past two years, compared with 7 percent of diabetics who were uninsured for less than a year and 5 percent of diabetics with health insurance (Ayanian et al., 2000). Adjusting results for the demographic characteristics of the national population, persons with diabetes who were uninsured for a year or longer were significantly less likely to have had a foot examination, a dilated eye examination, a cholesterol measurement, or a flu shot than were insured diabetics (Figure 3.1) (Ayanian et al., 2000).

End-Stage Renal Disease

Finding: Uninsured patients with end-stage renal disease begin dialysis at a later stage of disease than do insured patients and have poorer clinical measures of their condition at the time they begin dialysis.

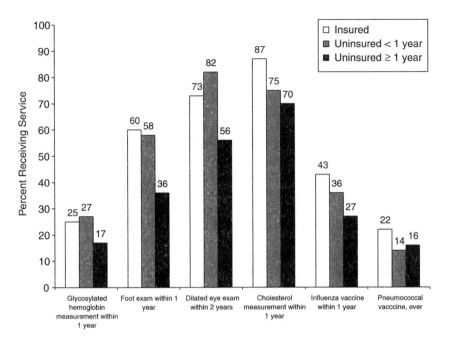

FIGURE 3.1 Diabetes management among insured and uninsured adults, ages 18–64. NOTE: Proportions adjusted to demographic characteristics of study cohort. SOURCE: Ayanian et al., 2000; Table 5.

Insurance status affects the timing and quality of care (Box 3.7) and may contribute to the longevity of dialysis patients, which is substantially lower than that of others of the same age (Obrador et al., 1999). The clinical goals for patients with kidney disease are to slow the progression of renal failure, manage complications, and prevent or manage comorbidities effectively. Although professional consensus about when dialysis should begin is not complete, there is agreement that the point in the progression of the disease at which dialysis begins affects patient outcomes (Kausz et al., 2000).

The Medicare ESRD program maintains extensive clinical and sociodemographic information on all dialysis patients, including information on patient health insurance status before beginning dialysis. This database provides opportunities to analyze the health care experience of all Americans who eventually develop ESRD, rather than just a sample of the population. One study that used this database analyzed the characteristics of 155,000 chronic dialysis patients who entered dialysis over a 27-month period between 1995 and 1997 (Obrador et al., 1999). This study found that uninsured patients were sicker at initiation of dialysis and less likely to have received erythropoietin (EPO) therapy than patients with any kind of insurance pre-ESRD. Uninsured patients also had an increased likelihood of hypoalbuminemia than those who had previously been privately insured (OR =

BOX 3.7
End-Stage Renal Disease

- In 2000, 90,000 people in the United States developed end-stage renal disease (kidney failure). Dialysis and transplantation are the two standard treatments. Approximately 300,000 patients are on dialysis and 80,000 have received kidney transplants (USRDS, 2001).
- The Medicare ESRD program provides coverage to 93 percent of those diagnosed with ESRD, and the U.S. Renal Data System collects clinical and sociodemographic information from dialysis and transplant centers on all ESRD patients, whether covered by Medicare or not.
- Hypoalbuminemia and low hematocrit (anemia) are factors related to poor dialysis outcomes, including cardiac failure and death. Anemia can be treated with erythropoietin (EPO) therapy prior to dialysis. Overall, 23 percent of beginning dialysis patients received EPO before they began dialysis (Obrador, 1999).
- Studies investigating the effects of insurance status on patients who develop ESRD examine prior therapy and clinical factors at the point at which dialysis is initiated.

1.37) and a greater likelihood of low hematocrit (<28 percent)[9] than the privately insured (OR = 1.34), after controlling for patients' sociodemographic and clinical characteristics, including comorbidities. Uninsured patients were also less likely than privately insured patients to have received EPO prior to dialysis (OR = 0.49) (Obrador et al., 1999). A second study based on the same data set found that patients without insurance were more likely to begin dialysis late[10] than were patients with any form of insurance (OR = 1.55) (Kausz et al., 2000).

Human Immunodeficiency Virus (HIV) Infection

Finding: Uninsured adults with HIV infection are less likely to receive highly effective medications that have been shown to improve survival.

A strong body of research about HIV infection confirms the findings of the general literature on insurance status and access to and use of services: uninsured adults diagnosed with HIV face greater delays in care than those with health insurance. They are less likely to receive regular care and drug therapy and are

---

[9]This standard of low hematocrit is below the hematocrit target range of 33–36 percent recommended by the National Kidney Foundation's Dialysis Outcomes Quality Initiative (NKF, 2001).

[10]In this study, "late initiation" is defined as glomerular filtration rate of serum creatinine of <5 ml/min per 1.73 m^2—a level substantially below both that recommended by the National Kidney Foundation (<10.5 ml/min) and the U.S. mean value at initiation (<7.1 ml/min) (Kausz et al., 2000).

> **BOX 3.8**
> **HIV Infection**
>
> • As of the beginning of 2000, the Centers for Disease Control and Prevention estimated that about 800,000 to 900,000 people were living with HIV infection or AIDS in the United States (CDC, 2001a).
> • In each of the years 1997, 1998, and 1999, between 40,000 and 50,000 new cases of AIDS were reported.
> • By 1996, combination antiretroviral therapy including protease inhibitors and nonnucleoside reverse transcriptase inhibitors, referred to as highly active antiretroviral therapies were becoming established as the treatment of choice for HIV infection (Carpenter et al., 1996). Largely as a result of these therapies, deaths among persons with AIDS dropped for the first time between 1996 and 1997 (by 42 percent) and declined 8 percent between 1998 and 1999 (CDC, 2001a).
> • About half of all adults with HIV infection see a provider at least once every six months (Bozzette et al., 1998).
> • Studies of HIV infection and health insurance examine a variety of health-related outcomes: general measures of access and utilization such as routine care visits and emergency department visits without hospitalization, delays between diagnosis and initiation of therapy, use of recommended drug therapies, and clinical outcomes such as CD4 lymphocyte counts.

more likely to go without needed care than patients with any kind of coverage (Cunningham et al., 1995, 1999; Katz et al., 1995; Shapiro et al., 1999).

A number of analyses have been based on national, longitudinal surveys evaluating access to care for persons with HIV infection (Niemcryk et al., 1998; Joyce et al., 1999; Shapiro et al., 1999; Andersen et al., 2000; Cunningham et al., 1999, 2000; Turner et al., 2000, Goldman et al., 2001).[11] These surveys allow assessment of the relationship between health insurance and access to care, use of services, receipt and timeliness of recommended therapies, and mortality as related to health insurance status. The research based on one of these surveys, the HIV Cost and Services Utilization Study (HCSUS), represents some of the most carefully designed studies of access to care and receipt of recommended therapies for specific conditions. In addition, there are several smaller, local studies based on

---

[11]The HIV Cost and Services Utilization Study (HSCUS), conducted by RAND and the Agency for Healthcare Research and Quality, was a probability sample of persons 18 years and older in the contiguous United States known to have HIV infection who had one visit for regular care (except in a military, prison, or emergency treatment facility) within a two-month period in 1996. Three rounds of interviews were conducted over a two-year period, 1996–1998, with between 2,267 and 2,864 subjects (Shapiro et al., 1999). The AIDS Costs and Utilization Survey, a predecessor study to HCSUS, with six waves over 18 months in 1991 and 1992, was not a probability sample (see Box 2.4 for further detail on these surveys).

hospital records or patient surveys (Katz et al., 1992, 1995; Bennett et al., 1995; Cunningham et al., 1995, 1996; Palacio et al, 1999; Sorvillo et al., 1999).

Access to a Regular Source of Care

Several studies suggest that the positive effects of health insurance for HIV-infected adults are achieved through the mechanism of having a regular source of care. Sorvillo and colleagues (1999) surveyed 339 HIV-positive adults in Los Angeles county in 1996–1997, and found that two-thirds of insured patients used protease inhibitors (PIs), while just half of uninsured patients were using them. When the site of care (private clinic, HMO, or public clinic) was included in a multivariable analysis, insurance status was no longer significantly related to receipt of PIs because of the concentration of uninsured patients in public clinics, which were less likely to prescribe PIs, especially at the beginning of the study period (Sorvillo et al., 1999).

Uninsured patients appear to face greater delays in beginning care following a diagnosis of HIV infection. In bivariate analysis of HCSUS data, uninsured patients were significantly more likely to have their first office visit more than three months after diagnosis with HIV than were privately insured patients (37 percent of uninsured patients had delays compared to 25 percent of privately insured patients in 1993; by 1995, those patients with delays decreased to 22 percent of uninsured patients and 14 percent of privately insured) (Turner et al., 2000). However, in a multivariable analysis, being uninsured was no longer a significant predictor of late initiation, while not having a regular source of care remained an important predictor (Turner et al., 2000).

Findings regarding emergency department (ED) use and hospitalization have changed over time. The most recent analysis, based on HCSUS, finds *greater* use of EDs, without hospitalization, and hospitalization more frequently than every six months for uninsured HIV patients (Shapiro et al., 1999), suggesting poorer access to other kinds of outpatient care. Studies based on earlier data report that uninsured patients had *lower* use of emergency rooms and hospitalization than either publicly or privately insured patients (Mor et al., 1992; Fleishman and Mor, 1993; Niemcryk et al., 1998; Joyce et al., 1999), suggesting poorer access even at high levels of acuity.

Receipt of Drug Therapies

Adults with HIV infection are more likely to receive effective drug therapies and to receive them earlier in the course of disease if they have health insurance. In an HCSUS analysis with extensive adjustments for sociodemographic and clinical factors, those without health insurance were much less likely to have ever received antiretroviral therapy (OR = 0.35) (Shapiro et al., 1999). Waiting times from diagnosis to the start of therapy with either PIs or nonnucleoside reverse transcriptase inhibitors, were 9.4 months for the privately insured, 12.4 months for Medicaid enrollees, and 13.9 months for uninsured patients (Shapiro et al., 2000).

Overall, many HIV-infected patients abandon recommended drug therapy over time. However, uninsured patients are more likely to stop drug therapy than are those with coverage. At the second follow-up interview of HCSUS respondents in 1997–1998, only half (53 percent) of all HIV-positive patients in care were receiving the recommended combination drug therapy, highly active antiretroviral therapy (HAART), although 71 percent had received HAART at some time in their treatment history (Cunningham et al., 2000). Uninsured patients were significantly less likely than privately insured patients with indemnity coverage (OR = 0.71) to be receiving HAART at the time of follow-up, indicating less appropriate care for uninsured patients with this disease (Cunningham et al., 2000).

Clinical Outcomes and Mortality

Studies of clinical outcomes for HIV patients present an evolving picture of both the efficacy of treatments and the impact of health insurance. A relatively early study of patients hospitalized with *Pneumocystis carinii* pneumonia (1987–1990) found that uninsured patients had a higher in-hospital mortality rate than did those with private insurance (OR = 1.49), and Medicaid patients had an even higher in-hospital mortality, relative to private patients (OR = 2.1) (Bennett et al., 1995). Another early and small study (96 patients in one university clinic) found that patients with private insurance had significantly lower CD4 lymphocyte counts (a worse outcome) than either uninsured or Medicaid patients (who had the highest counts), when first treated at the clinic (Katz et al., 1992). The authors hypothesize that some relatively healthy patients with private health insurance coverage may have been reluctant to use it and thus reported their status as uninsured.

More recently, an analysis based on HCSUS examined the mortality experience of insured and uninsured HIV-infected adults and found that having health insurance of any kind reduced the risk of dying within six months of being surveyed between 71 and 85 percent, when severity of illness (measured by CD4 lymphocyte count) and sociodemographic characteristics were controlled (Goldman et al., 2001). The greater reduction in mortality risk (85 percent) was estimated for a surviving subset (2,466 participants) of the original 1996 sample of 2,864 participants a year later, when HAART was in wider use and was reducing mortality among HIV patients who used it. This impact of health insurance on mortality for HIV-infected adults within a short follow-up period, six months, demonstrates how sensitive health outcomes can be to coverage when it facilitates receipt of effective therapy.

BOX 3.9
Mental Illness

• About 38 million people ages 18 and older are estimated to have a single mental disorder of any severity or both a mental and an addictive disorder in a given year (Narrow et al., 2002).
• The most common conditions fall into the broad categories of schizophrenia, affective disorders (including major depression and bipolar or manic–depressive illness), and anxiety disorders (typically includes panic disorder, obsessive–compulsive disorder, posttraumatic stress disorder, and phobia).
• Schizophrenia has been estimated to affect about 2 million Americans in any one year and about 9 million adults experience a major depressive episode in any year, including an estimated 1 million with manic-depressive (bipolar) disorder (Narrow et al., 2002). Anxiety disorders affect an estimated 24 million Americans annually (Narrow et al., 2002).
• Only 25 percent of people who have a mental disorder obtain diagnosis and treatment from the health care system, in contrast to 60–80 percent of those with heart disease (USDHHS, 2000).
• Evidence-based practice guidelines for depression endorse antidepressant medications and cognitive–behavioral or interpersonal psychotherapies (AHCPR, 1993; U.S. Department of Veterans Affairs, 1993; Schulberg et al., 1998).
• Studies of the effects of health insurance status on care and outcomes for mental illnesses examine receipt of any services for the condition, guideline-concordant care, and care within the mental health sector.

Mental Illness

Finding: Health insurance that covers any mental health treatment is associated with the receipt of mental health care and with care consistent with clinical practice guidelines from both general medical and specialty mental health providers.

Mental disorders or illnesses are health conditions that are characterized by changes in thinking, mood, or behavior. They are often chronic conditions but may also occur as single or infrequent episodes over a lifetime. Mental illnesses represent a major source of disability in the United States that is often underestimated by the public and health care professionals alike (USDHHS, 2000). In industrialized economies, mental illness is equivalent to heart disease and cancer in terms of its impact on disability (Murray and Lopez, 1996).

Despite the differential treatment of mental health services in both public and private insurance plans, the studies reviewed by the Committee document a positive association between health insurance coverage and more appropriate care for mental illnesses (Box 3.9). Health insurance plans and programs historically have excluded services related to treatment for mental illness, strictly limited coverage of mental health services, and administered mental health benefits separately from other kinds of medical care. Thus, studies that attempt to measure the effects of health insurance status on health care and outcomes for mental illnesses may be affected by the diversity of health insurance benefits and of cost sharing and administrative requirements for these services and conditions. Variability in benefits among health insurance plans and types of insurance complicates the interpretation of all observational studies of health insurance effects but poses a particular problem vis–a–vis mental health. (See the discussion of measurement bias in Chapter 2.)

The use of mental health services in both the general and specialty mental health sectors by adults is positively associated with health insurance coverage (Cooper-Patrick et al., 1999; Wang et al., 2000; Young et al., 2001). Between 1987 and 1997, the overall rate of treatment for depression among American adults under age 65 tripled from 1 person per 100 to 3.2 persons per 100, yet the treatment rate among those without health insurance was half that of the overall population rate in 1997, 1.5 persons treated per 100 population (Olfson et al., 2002). A longitudinal, community-based study in Baltimore, Maryland, between 1981 and 1996 documented increased use of mental health services over this period (Cooper-Patrick et al., 1999). Analyzing the experience of African Americans and whites separately, the authors found that for African Americans specifically, this increase was achieved predominantly with services provided in the general medical sector. For both African Americans and whites, being uninsured reduced the likelihood of receiving any mental health services.

At the same time, insurance coverage for adults with mental illness is less stable than average for those without this condition (Sturm and Wells, 2000; Rabinowitz et al., 2001). In a recent (1998) follow-up survey of participants in the Community Tracking Study, those who reported having symptoms of mental disorders were found to be more likely to lose coverage within a year following their diagnosis than those without a mental disorder (Sturm and Wells, 2000). As discussed below, those with severe mental illness also experience transitions in insurance coverage, frequently ending up with public program coverage (Rabinowitz et al., 2001).

The findings reported below are grouped into those for depression and anxiety disorders and those for severe mental illnesses. Depression and anxiety disorders are often treatable in the general medical sector and primarily require outpatient services. Severe mental illnesses (schizophrenia, other psychoses, and bipolar depression) require the attention of specialty mental health professionals and may require inpatient and other forms of more extensive services (e.g., partial or day hospitalization). Public health insurance, both Medicare and Medicaid, is an important source of coverage for specialty mental health services for those disabled by severe mental illness (SMI).

Depression and Anxiety Disorders

Receipt of appropriate (guideline-concordant) care for depression is associated with improved functional outcomes at two years (Sturm and Wells, 1995).

Health insurance coverage specifically for mental health services is associated with an increased likelihood of receiving such care. Two studies support this claim.

The first, a nationally representative study of three prevalent disorders—depression, panic disorder, and generalized anxiety disorder—investigated the contribution of insurance coverage and health care utilization to guideline-concordant treatment (Wang et al., 2000). Mental health diagnoses were determined in a structured interview using a well-defined operational definition of mental health care over the previous 12 months. Treatment criteria included the combination of a prescription medication for depression or anxiety from a general medical doctor or a psychiatrist in addition to at least four visits to the same type of provider or, where medication was not prescribed, a minimum of eight visits to either a psychiatrist or a mental health specialist (Wang et al., 2000). A multivariable analysis estimated the effects of sociodemographic characteristics, various measures of clinical status including a measure of mental illness severity, insurance coverage for mental health visits, number and reasons for use of general medical services, other medications, and alternative therapies. Patients diagnosed with depression, panic disorder, or a generalized anxiety disorder who had no health insurance coverage for mental health visits were less likely to receive any mental health services (OR = 0.43). They were also less likely to receive guideline-concordant care in the general medical sector (OR = 0.24) or in the mental health treatment sector (OR = 0.36) (Wang et al., 2000).

A second study of adults with a probable 12-month diagnosis of depression or anxiety examined factors associated with receipt of appropriate care (psychiatric medication and counseling) (Young et al, 2001): 1,636 respondents were identified as having one or more depressive or anxiety disorders based on a structured diagnostic interview. Respondents with a depressive or anxiety disorder who had more education and a greater number of medical disorders were more likely to have had contact with providers than those with less education and fewer medical conditions. Those with no health insurance were less likely to have had any provider contact than were those with any form of health insurance (OR = 0.46). However, for those receiving any care, insurance status was not related to receipt of appropriate care (Young et al., 2001). These findings suggest that health insurance alone may not ensure appropriate mental health care.

Severe Mental Illness

Uninsured adults with severe mental illnesses are less likely to receive appropriate care than are those with coverage and may experience delays in receiving services until they gain public insurance.

In a study using the same sample and survey as that used by Young and colleagues, McAlpine and Mechanic (2001) investigated the association of current insurance coverage and specialty mental health utilization within the past 12 months (i.e., visits to a psychiatrist or psychologist, hospital admission, or emergency room visit for an emotional or substance use problem) for SMI. Two diagnostic indices, including a global measure of mental health, measured the need for care. Potential confounding factors such as physical symptoms and degree of dangerousness and disruptiveness were also measured. One in five respondents identified with an SMI was uninsured. Among persons with SMI, those without health insurance were far less likely to use specialty mental health services than those with Medicare or Medicaid (OR = 0.17) (McAlpine and Mechanic, 2000).

Individuals with SMIs typically lack insurance at the time of hospitalization (Rabinowitz et al., 2001). An important question regarding insurance coverage in this patient population is whether a first hospitalization for SMI results in a change in insurance status and whether such a change influences subsequent mental health care. Rabinowitz and colleagues followed the progress of 443 individuals enrolled in a county mental health project to determine whether changes in coverage followed first admission for psychosis and the association between type of insurance coverage and future care. Overall, the proportion of patients with no insurance 24 months after hospitalization decreased from 42 percent at baseline to 21 percent as a result of enrollment in public insurance programs. Men were more likely to remain uninsured than were women. The total number of days of care received (inpatient, outpatient, day hospital) was significantly higher for the publicly insured group compared to both those with private insurance and those with no insurance during the first 6 months after initial hospitalization and over the entire 24-month period. Uninsured patients with SMI were much less likely to receive outpatient care after hospitalization than patients with Medicaid or Medicare (OR = 0.24) and also less likely than those with private health insurance to receive outpatient care subsequent to hospitalization (OR = 0.56) (Rabinowitz et al., 2001).

An earlier study using the same data also reported an association between health insurance and receipt of mental health services prior to a first admission for psychotic disorder (Rabinowitz et al., 1998). Forty-four percent of patients (n = 525) were uninsured at first admission. Uninsured patients were less likely than those with private insurance to have had

- any mental health treatment prior to admission (OR = 0.53),
- specific psychotherapeutic contact (OR = 0.43),
- voluntary admission (OR = 0.56),
- less than three months between onset of psychosis and admission (OR = 0.56)

and were less likely to have been admitted to a community (versus public) hospital (OR = 0.14) (Rabinowitz et al., 1998). Uninsured patients were also less likely than those with either Medicaid or Medicare to have received antipsychotic medication (OR = 0.4), had voluntary admission (OR = 0.53), and be admitted to a community hospital (OR = 0.33).

HOSPITAL-BASED CARE

Finding: Uninsured patients who are hospitalized for a range of conditions experience higher rates of death in the hospital, receive fewer services, and are more likely to experience an adverse medical event due to negligence than are insured patients.

Americans assume and expect that hospital-based care for serious and emergency conditions is available to everyone, regardless of health insurance coverage, while recognizing that uninsured patients may be limited to treatment at public or otherwise designated "safety-net" hospitals (IOM, 2001a). Professional and institutional standards of practice grounded in ethics, law, and licensure dictate that the care received by all patients, regardless of financial or insurance status, be of equal and high quality. Yet studies of hospital-based care conducted over the past two decades have documented differences in the services received by insured and uninsured patients, differences in the quality of their care (sometimes but not always related to the site of care), and differences in patient outcomes such as in-hospital mortality rates.[12]

One of the most comprehensive of these studies of hospitalization analyzed more than 592,000 hospital discharge abstracts in 1987 (Hadley et al., 1991). The authors report that for adults ages 18–65, uninsured hospital inpatients had a significantly higher risk of dying in the hospital than their privately insured counterparts in 8 of 12 age–sex–race-specific population cohorts (relative risks ranged from 1.1 for black women ages 50–64 to 3.2 for black men ages 35–49). This analysis adjusted for patient condition on admission to the hospital. Uninsured patients were also less likely to receive endoscopic procedures in the hospital than privately insured patients, and when they did receive these diagnostic services, the resultant pathology reports were more likely to be abnormal (OR = 1.56) (Hadley et al., 1991).

This study by Hadley and colleagues also examined the relative resource use (length of stay) of uninsured hospital patients compared to privately insured patients and found that for conditions that afford high discretion in treatment decisions (e.g., tonsillitis, bronchitis, hernia), uninsured patients had significantly shorter lengths of stay (Hadley et al., 1991). However, for diagnoses that afford little discretion in treatment (e.g., gastrointestinal hemorrhage, congestive heart failure), lengths of stay were not significantly different for uninsured and privately insured patients, although uninsured patients tended to have shorter stays. This underscores the possibility that when uninsured patients are found to receive

---

[12]Older studies that examine hospital-based care and outcomes according to insurance status across a range of diagnoses are summarized in Appendix B. The results of these studies are consistent with the findings discussed in text; however, many are based on hospital records that may be less relevant to the current hospital practice environment.

fewer services than insured patients, it may be the result of overtreatment of patients with insurance, rather than undertreatment of those without coverage.

In addition to differences in the resources devoted to the care of insured and uninsured patients, the quality of the care provided may differ. One study of more than 30,000 hospital medical records in 51 hospitals in New York State for 1984 found that the proportion of adverse medical events due to negligence was substantially greater among patients without health insurance than among privately insured patients (OR = 2.35), while the experience of Medicaid patients did not differ significantly from that of the privately insured population (Burstin et al., 1992). This increased risk for uninsured patients was attributable only in part to receiving care more frequently in emergency departments, which generally were found to have higher rates of adverse events.

Because most studies of hospital-based care and outcomes are observational, including only those who literally "show up" for care, and because appropriateness criteria are not available for many conditions, some of the strongest research on health insurance effects involves studies of specific conditions. Studies of certain conditions are less likely to be compromised by nonrandom or unrepresentative samples (selection bias) simply because a larger proportion of the population of interest—namely, acutely ill adults—is likely to be captured in the hospital-based study population. Furthermore, condition-specific studies are more likely to include evidence-based criteria for judging the appropriateness of care.

The following two sections consider research that has examined the effect of health insurance on care and outcomes for patients with (1) emergency conditions and traumatic injuries and (2) cardiovascular disease. For both categories, selection bias among those reaching treatment is minimized, and appropriateness guidelines and outcomes criteria (e.g., mortality) are definitive. Traumatic injuries (specifically automobile accidents), for example, reduce some of the unmeasured differences in propensity to seek care between insured and uninsured patients (Doyle, 2001). Another area of hospital-based services for which there is sufficient professional consensus about appropriate treatment is the use of angiography and revascularization procedures following acute myocardial infarction (AMI) or heart attack, at least for a subset of patients with severe coronary artery disease.[13]

Emergency and Trauma Care

Finding: Uninsured persons with traumatic injuries are less likely to be admitted to the hospital, receive fewer services when admitted, and are more likely to die than insured trauma victims.

---

[13]See Leape et al. (1999) for a description of the RAND methodology for determining appropriateness and its application to developing criteria for revascularization procedures.

BOX 3.10
Trauma

• Throughout the United States in 1997, approximately 34.4 million episodes of injury and poisoning received medical attention and 40.9 million injuries and poisonings were reported as a result (Warner et al., 2000).
• For injury-related deaths, 43 percent involved automobiles or traffic, more than three times as many deaths as the second most-common cause, falls (13 percent) (NCHS, 2001). Traffic-related injuries comprised almost 11 percent of all injuries (McCaig and Burt, 2001).
• There were approximately 102.8 million visits to hospital EDs during 1999, of which 13 percent resulted in admission to the hospital (McCaig and Burt, 2001). Almost 37 percent of all ED visits were for injuries (McCaig and Burt, 2001; Warner et al., 2000).
• Medical screening, stabilization of an acute or life-threatening condition, and transfer are guaranteed universally by the federal Emergency Medical Treatment and Active Labor Act of 1986.
• Studies of health insurance status, EDs, and traumatic injury have examined outcomes such as severity-adjusted admissions rates, services and resource use, interhospital transfers, and mortality.

Two studies based on large, statewide data sets have found substantial and significant differences in the risk of dying for insured and uninsured trauma patients (Box 3.10) who were admitted to hospitals as emergencies. Doyle (2001) analyzed more than 10,000 police reports of auto accidents linked to hospital records maintained by Wisconsin over 1992–1997 to ascertain the care received and the mortality of insured and uninsured crash victims. After controlling for personal, crash, and hospital characteristics, it was found that uninsured accident victims received 20 percent less care, as measured by hospital charges and length of stay, and had a 37 percent higher mortality rate than did privately insured accident victims (5.2 percent versus 3.8 percent, respectively) (Doyle, 2001). The authors conclude that these differences are attributable to provider response to insurance status because extensive patient characteristics were accounted for in the analysis and because unmeasured patient characteristics that might influence these outcomes were unlikely to be related to patients' health insurance status.

Haas and Goldman (1994) evaluated the treatment experience and mortality of more than 15,000 insured and uninsured trauma patients admitted to hospitals on an emergency basis in Massachusetts in 1990. Adjusting the data for injury severity and comorbidities as well as for age, sex, and race, the authors found that uninsured trauma patients received less care and had higher in-hospital mortality than did patients with private insurance or Medicaid. Uninsured patients were just as likely to receive care in an intensive care unit (ICU) as privately insured trauma patients but were less likely to undergo an operative procedure (OR = 0.68) or to receive physical therapy (OR = 0.61). Uninsured patients were much more likely than privately insured patients to die in the hospital (OR = 2.15) (Haas and Goldman, 1994). The differences in services and mortality experience between Medicaid and privately insured patients were small and were not statistically significant.

Other studies of emergency department use and admissions and care for traumatic injuries shed some light on patient behavior and institutional responses related to health insurance status. Both lacking health insurance and not having a regular source of care have been found in surveys of patients who eventually do arrive at an ED to be related to delays in seeking care (Ell et al., 1994; Rucker et al., 2001). Braveman and colleagues (1994) examined hospital discharge records of more than 91,000 adults diagnosed with acute appendicitis in California hospitals between 1984 and 1989. They found that the risk of a ruptured appendix was 50 percent higher for both uninsured and Medicaid patients, than for privately insured patients in prepaid plans, in an analysis that controlled for age, sex, race, psychiatric diagnoses, diabetes, and hospital characteristics. Admission to a public hospital also was associated with rupture, as were diagnoses of psychiatric illness or diabetes (Braveman et al., 1994). The authors hypothesized that both Medicaid and uninsured patients incurred avoidable delays before seeking care for appendicitis.

Three separate studies that analyzed Medicaid and uninsured trauma patients together report mixed findings regarding patient outcomes and hospital care. Rhee and colleagues (1997) examined patient information for more than 2,800 persons hospitalized at a Level 1 trauma center after a motor vehicle crash in Seattle, Washington, between 1990 and 1993.[14] This study found no significant differences in mortality, hospital charges, or length of stay (LOS) between privately insured patients and those who either had Medicaid coverage or were uninsured, except for patients who ultimately were transferred to a long-term care or rehabilitation facility. In the case of patients awaiting transfer, those with Medicaid or no insurance had an adjusted LOS that was 11 percent longer than privately insured patients (Rhee et al., 1997). The authors speculate that the similarity in treatment and outcomes for patients of different insurance status could be due to the mission of the public, Level 1 trauma center to which they were admitted, which was to serve the entire state population needing that level of care and act as a provider of last resort for uninsured patients. Because this study did not differentiate results for Medicaid and uninsured patients, it provides less informa-

---

[14]The American College of Surgeons designates hospital EDs as trauma centers based on qualifying criteria related to staffing, resources, and services. There are four designations: Level 1, the most stringent requirements, for providing tertiary care on a regional basis; Level 2, similar services to a Level 1 center but without clinical research and prevention activities; Level 3, presence of emergency services, often in a rural area, with fewer specialized services and resources than Level 1 or 2 centers; and Level 4, usually in a rural area, describing hospitals and clinics that serve a triage function (Bonnie et al., 1999).

tion about outcomes for uninsured patients than studies that analyze these groups separately.

Uninsured trauma patients may also be treated differently from insured patients in interhospital transfer decisions. Using Washington State trauma registry information, Nathens and colleagues (2001) identified 2,008 trauma patients between 16 and 64 years of age injured in King County (Seattle) and originally transported to one of seven Level 3 or 4 trauma centers in the county between 1995 and 1999. Adjusting for age, sex, type of injury, and injury severity, they looked at independent predictors of transfer to the Level 1 trauma center in the county—a public, safety-net hospital, and estimated that patients who either had Medicaid or were uninsured were more than twice as likely to be transferred to the higher level facility than were privately insured patients (OR = 2.4) and that many of these transferred patients had low injury severity scores (ISS).[15] The authors conclude that this "payer-based triage" may undermine the effectiveness of Level 1 trauma centers in serving the more critically injured patients by diverting resources to patients who could have been treated appropriately in their original hospital (Nathens et al., 2001).

Finally, the differences found between uninsured and insured patients in highly discretionary cases may reflect overtreatment of those with health insurance rather than undertreatment of uninsured patients. Svenson and Spurlock (2001) evaluated the experience of more than 8,500 patients with head injuries treated in four Kentucky hospitals between 1995 and 1997. For those with less severe head injuries (lacerations, contusion, or concussion), uninsured patients were substantially less likely than privately insured patients to be admitted to the hospital (OR = 0.14 for laceration, 0.38 for contusion or concussion). The likelihood of admission for Medicaid was also substantially lower than for privately insured patients, but not as low as for uninsured patients (ORs = 0.33 and 0.45, respectively). Little difference was found in hospital admissions for more severe head injuries among patients with different insurance status. The authors were unable to determine whether the differences in admissions for less severe head trauma are due to undertreatment of uninsured and Medicaid patients or overtreatment of privately insured patients (Svenson and Spurlock, 2001).

Cardiovascular Disease

Finding: Uninsured patients with acute cardiovascular disease are less likely to be admitted to a hospital that performs angiography or revascularization procedures, are less likely to receive these diagnostic and treatment procedures, and are more likely to die in the short term.

---

[15]The authors designated an ISS of <16 as "minimal to moderate injury" and >16 as more severe. Overall, 59 percent of transferred patients had an ISS of <9.

> **BOX 3.11**
> **Coronary Artery Disease**
>
> • In 2001, an estimated 1.1 million Americans suffered a diagnosed heart attack. An estimated 7.3 million Americans have a history of AMI (American Heart Association, 2001).
> • During 1998, coronary heart disease accounted for about 460,000 deaths; AMI was responsible for more than 200,000 of these deaths (CDC, 2001b).
> • Approximately 1.3 million diagnostic cardiac catheterizations (angiography) were performed in 1998. In the same year, about 550,000 coronary artery bypass graft (CABG) surgeries were performed on 336,000 patients, and about 530,000 patients received percutaneous transluminal coronary angioplasty (PTCA). In each case, roughly half of the patients receiving the service were younger than 65 (American Heart Association, 2001).
> • Studies of health insurance status and its effects on diagnosis, treatment, and outcomes for cardiovascular disease have examined overall rates of diagnostic and treatment services (cardiac catheterization, CABG, PTCA), rates for hospitalized post-AMI patients for whom they are deemed nondiscretionary, and inpatient and 30-day posthospitalization mortality.

Finding: Health insurance reduces the disparity in receipt of these services by members of racial and ethnic minority groups.

Health insurance is positively associated with receipt of hospital-based treatments for cardiovascular disease (specifically, coronary artery disease) and with lower patient mortality (Box 3.11). One meta-analysis has credited medical advances in the treatment of cardiovascular disease, including hospital-based care following AMI, with roughly half of the reduction in post-AMI mortality between 1975 and 1995 (with a range of 20 to 85 percent) (Cutler et al., 1998). Some of the most recent studies have used appropriateness criteria to identify when a given procedure is considered necessary according to professional consensus, reducing the chances that differences in rates between uninsured and insured patients are a result of overtreatment of the insured population (i.e., Sada et al.,1998; Leape et al., 1999).

Mortality

Five studies that examined the mortality experience of patients hospitalized for cardiovascular disease (including AMI, angina, and chest pain) reported higher in-hospital or 30-day posthospitalization mortality for uninsured patients (Young and Cohen, 1991; Blustein et al., 1995; Kreindel et al., 1997; Sada et al., 1998; Canto et al., 2000).

The first study, of about 5,000 patients admitted on an emergency basis for AMI in 1987, found that uninsured patients were more likely to die within 30 days of admission than privately insured patients (OR = 1.5) (Young and Cohen, 1991). In a second study, Blustein and colleagues (1995) examined records for 5,800 patients under 65 who were admitted to California hospitals for AMI in 1991 and found that uninsured patients were more likely to die in the hospital than privately insured patients (OR = 1.9) and still had an increased risk of dying after adjusting for receipt of a revascularization procedure (OR = 1.7). Finally, a study in a single Massachusetts community of 3,700 patients hospitalized for AMI between 1986 and 1993 reported that uninsured patients had a slight, but statistically insignificant greater in-hospital mortality than privately insured patients (OR = 1.2, CI: 0.6–2.4) (Kreindel et al., 1997).

Two larger studies that used more recent data (1994–1996) from the National Registry of Myocardial Infarction reported higher in-hospital mortality for uninsured than for privately insured patients. In the first, Sada and colleagues (1998) reviewed records for 17,600 patients under age 65 who were admitted to hospital for AMI and found that uninsured patients had an in-hospital mortality rate of 5.4 percent, compared with 3.8 percent for private FFS patients and 3.9 percent for private HMO patients. Medicaid patients had the highest in-hospital mortality rate, 8.9 percent. In a model that adjusted for demographic and clinical factors, the likelihood of uninsured patients dying in the hospital was still higher but was not statistically significantly different from that of privately insured patients (OR = 1.2, CI: 0.8–1.6) (Sada et al, 1998). The second national study examined records for more than 332,000 patients admitted with AMI and found that after adjusting for demographics, prior disease history, and clinical characteristics, uninsured patients were more likely to die in the hospital than privately insured FFS patients (OR = 1.29) (Canto et al., 2000). The mortality experience of Medicaid patients was the same as that of uninsured patients.

Only one study, a review of hospital records of 1,556 patients undergoing coronary artery bypass graft surgery in a single Louisiana teaching hospital, found that uninsured patients had better long-term survival than did insured patients (Mancini et al., 2001). However, this study did not control for age or characteristics of the patients. The average age of uninsured patients at the time of surgery was 55, and of insured patients, 65 years. Furthermore, only 7 percent of the insured study population had private insurance, so the population was not representative of the insured population at large.

Coronary Procedures

The body of research on the use of specific procedures to diagnose and treat cardiovascular disease as a function of the insurance status of the patient consistently reports differences in utilization, with uninsured patients generally less likely to receive coronary angiography, CABG, or percutaneous transluminal coronary angioplasty (PTCA) than privately insured patients (Young and Cohen, 1991; Blustein et al., 1995; Kuykendall et al., 1995; Sada et al., 1998; Leape et al., 1999; Canto et al., 2000; Daumit et al., 2000). However, only some of these studies applied appropriateness criteria to identify cases in which the use of these procedures was considered nondiscretionary or necessary. In the studies that examined overall utilization rates, the differences found by insurance status could be attributed to overutilization as well as underutilization.

Angiography (cardiac catheterization) is an invasive diagnostic procedure that provides information to guide decisions about subsequent treatment options, including revascularization procedures. Sada and colleagues (1998) applied the criteria of the American College of Cardiology and American Heart Association Joint Task Force to a national data set of 17,600 myocardial infarction patients under 65 to identify nondiscretionary angiography for revascularization candidates considered to be at high risk. They estimated that in hospitals providing these cardiac procedures, patients with private FFS coverage who were deemed high-risk and for whom angiography was nondiscretionary were more likely than similarly high-risk uninsured patients or Medicaid patients to receive angiography. Among high-risk FFS patients, 84 percent received this service compared to 73 percent of high-risk uninsured patients and 60 percent of similar Medicaid patients (Sada et al., 1998).

Revascularization procedures (either CABG or PTCA) following a heart attack are also more likely to be performed on insured than uninsured patients. In two studies, uninsured patients were less likely to receive revascularization (either CABG or PTCA) than privately insured FFS patients (OR = 0.6 in the 1991 study and 0.8 in the 2000 study) (Young and Cohen, 1991; Canto et al., 2000). Blustein and colleagues (1995) and Kuykendall and colleagues (1995) reported similar comparative findings regarding the revascularization of uninsured and privately insured patients (ORs in these studies ranged from 0.4 to 0.6).

InterHospital Transfers to Receive Services. For patients with AMI, health insurance facilitates access to hospitals that perform angiography and revascularization, whether admission is initial or by means of an interhospital transfer (Blustein et al., 1995; Canto et al., 1999; Leape et al., 1999).

In a study of California hospital admissions for AMI, Blustein and colleagues (1995) found that uninsured patients were less likely than privately insured patients to be admitted initially to a hospital that offered revascularization and much less likely to be transferred if admitted initially to one that did not (ORs = 0.71 and 0.42, respectively).

Leape and colleagues (1999) reviewed 631 records for patients who had received angiography and subsequently met expert panel criteria for necessary revascularization. Overall, 74 percent of patients meeting these criteria received revascularization. Leape et al. found that in hospitals that also performed CABG and PTCA, there were no differences in rates of revascularization for patients with different insurance status. However, for patients initially hospitalized in facilities that did *not* perform CABG and PTCA, who required a transfer to another hospital to receive revascularization, the rates differed significantly by insurance status: 91 percent of Medicare patients, 82 percent of privately insured patients, 75 percent of Medicaid patients, and just 52 percent of uninsured patients received this indicated surgery (Leape et al., 1999).

Insurance Status and Racial and Gender Disparities. Health insurance has been shown to lessen disparities in the care for cardiovascular disease received by men compared to women and among members of racial and ethnic groups (Carlisle et al., 1997; Daumit et al., 1999, 2000).

An analysis of more than 100,000 hospital discharges with a principal diagnosis of cardiovascular disease in Los Angeles County between 1986 and 1988 revealed significant differences in rates of angiography, CABG, and PTCA between *uninsured* African-American and white patients but not between members of these ethnic groups who were privately insured (Carlisle et al., 1997). In a multivariate analysis that controlled for demographic and clinical characteristics and hospital procedure volume, the odds ratios for uninsured African Americans to receive one of these services compared with uninsured whites ranged from 0.33 to 0.5 (Carlisle et al., 1997).

A longitudinal study with a seven-year follow-up of a national random sample of patients who initially became eligible for the Medicare ESRD program in 1986 or 1987 found that once uninsured patients qualified for ESRD benefits, pronounced disparities by gender or race in their likelihood of receiving either angiography, CABG, or PTCA were eliminated (Daumit et al., 1999, 2000). In the period prior to qualifying for Medicare, uninsured African Americans were far less likely than uninsured whites to undergo a cardiac procedure (OR = 0.07) (Daumit et al., 1999). Uninsured women were also less likely than uninsured men to receive a cardiac procedure before qualifying for Medicare (OR = 0.4), and uninsured men were much less likely than men with private insurance to receive one (OR = 0.47) (Daumit et al., 2000). In the case of both race and gender, differences in the receipt of these cardiac procedures were eliminated after gaining Medicare ESRD coverage.

GENERAL HEALTH OUTCOMES

Finding: Longitudinal population-based studies of the mortality of uninsured and privately insured adults reveal a higher risk of dying for those who were uninsured at baseline than for those who initially had private coverage.

Finding: Relatively short (one- to four-year) longitudinal studies document relatively greater decreases in general health status measures for uninsured adults and for those who lost insurance coverage during the period studied than for those with continuous coverage.

This chapter concludes with a review of the studies evaluating the overall health status and mortality experience of insured and uninsured populations. Assessments of general health outcomes such as self-reported health status and mortality or survival rates for uninsured adults under 65 compared to those with some form of health insurance (i.e., employment-sponsored, Medicaid, Medicare, individually purchased policies), present researchers with even greater challenges of analytic adjustment than those encountered in studies of specific health conditions. Not only might health insurance affect health status, but health status can affect health insurance status. Thus, it is difficult to interpret cross-sectional studies of health insurance and health status. However, several well-designed longitudinal studies with extensive analytic adjustments for covariates have found higher mortality and worse overall functional and health status among uninsured adults than among otherwise similar insured adults.

Mortality

Two studies provide evidence that uninsured adults are more likely to die prematurely than are their privately insured counterparts.

Franks and colleagues (1993a) followed a national cohort of 4,700 adults age 25 or older for 13 to 17 years who, at the baseline interview, were either privately insured or uninsured. At the end of the follow-up period (1987), about twice as many participants who were uninsured at the time of the first interview had died as had those with private health insurance (18.4 percent compared with 9.6 percent). Controlling for sociodemographic characteristics, health examination findings, self-reported health status, and health behaviors, the risk of death for adults who initially were uninsured was 25 percent greater than for those who had private health insurance at the time of the initial interview (mortality hazard ratio = 1.25, CI: 1.00–1.55). The magnitude of this independent health insurance effect on mortality risk was comparable to that of being unemployed, to lacking a high school diploma, or to being in the lowest income category (Franks et al., 1993a).[16] Because insurance status was measured only at the initial interview and thus did not reflect the subjects' cumulative insurance experience over the 13–17 year follow-up period, the difference found in mortality between uninsured and privately insured persons most likely is an underestimate of differences in the mortality experience of those who are continuously uninsured and those who are continuously insured.

A study by Sorlie and colleagues (1994) tracked the mortality experience of 148,000 adults between 25 and 65 years of age until 1987, a two- to five-year follow-up period. After adjusting for age and income, this study found that uninsured white men had a 20 percent higher risk of dying than white men with

---

[16]The lowest income category included those with a family income of less than $7,000 at the initial interview (1971–1975).

employment-based health insurance. Uninsured black men and white women each had a 50 percent higher mortality risk than their counterparts with employment-based coverage (Sorlie et al., 1994). Among black women, insurance was not statistically associated with mortality. The authors also examined the mortality experience of insured and uninsured *employed* white men and women, adjusted for age and income. (Because of small sample size, they did not perform this analysis for black men and women.)   Uninsured employed white men had a 30 percent greater risk of dying than their working counterparts with health insurance, and uninsured employed white women had a 20 percent greater risk over two to five years than their counterparts with health insurance (Sorlie et al., 1994).

Loss of Coverage and Changes in Health Status Over Time

Persons who lose health insurance have been found to experience declines in their health status. Longitudinal studies that follow a cohort of individuals over time can provide a "before-and-after" picture of health status, comparing a group that maintained coverage with one that lost it. Such a design helps to minimize the possibility that unmeasured factors that vary along with health insurance status account for differences in health, a competing hypothesis that cannot be eliminated in cross-sectional studies.

Lurie and colleagues (1984, 1986) took advantage of a natural experiment in the mid-1980s when California eliminated Medi-Cal coverage for a group of medically indigent adults. Following matched cohorts of adults seen at an internal medicine practice at a university clinic who either maintained or lost Medi-Cal coverage, the authors found that the patients who lost coverage reported significant decreases in perceived overall health at both six months and a year later, unlike those who maintained coverage. As discussed earlier in this chapter, participants in this study with hypertension who lost coverage also experienced worsening blood pressure control, while those who maintained coverage did not.

Like those with chronic health conditions, adults in late middle age are particularly susceptible to deteriorations of function and health status if they lack or lose health insurance coverage. Baker and colleagues (2001) followed a group of more than 7,500 participants in the longitudinal Health and Retirement Survey (adults ages 51 to 61 at the outset) between 1992 and 1996. The authors compared three groups:

1. those who were *continuously insured* over the first two years (measured in 1992 and 1994);

2. those who were *continuously without insurance* over that period; and

3. those who were *intermittently uninsured*, defined as those who lacked health insurance either in 1992 or in 1994, but not at both times (Baker et al., 2001).

Of those who were continuously uninsured, 22 percent had a major decline[17] in self-reported health, 16 percent of the intermittently uninsured experienced a major decline, and 8 percent of the continuously insured reported a major decline in health. In an analysis that controlled for sociodemographic characteristics, pre-existing medical conditions, and health behaviors, the authors estimated a 60 percent greater risk of a major decline in health for continuously uninsured persons and a 40 percent greater risk for intermittently insured persons, as compared with continuously insured persons. Continuously or intermittently uninsured persons also had a 20 to 25 percent greater risk of developing a new difficulty in walking or climbing stairs than did those who were continuously insured (Baker et al., 2001).

Cross-Sectional Studies of Health Status

Cross-sectional studies based on large national population surveys (Medical Expenditure Panel Survey [MEPS], National Medical Expenditure Survey [NMES], and Behavioral Risk Factor Surveillance System, provide snapshots of the subjective or self-reported health status of populations according to insurance status. These surveys report worse health status among those without insurance than among those with coverage. Two large studies with careful and extensive analytic adjustments for covarying personal characteristics are presented here.

Franks and colleagues (1993b) examined the relationship between health insurance status and subjective health across several dimensions, including a general health perceptions scale, physical and role functions, and mental health, for 12,000 adults ages 25 through 64. The authors compared participants who had private health insurance for an entire year with those who had been without health insurance the entire year. In an analysis that controlled for age, sex, race, education, presence of a medical condition, and attitude toward medical care and insurance, uninsured adults had significantly lower subjective health scores across all dimensions. The effect on these measures of health of being uninsured was greater for lower-income persons than for those in families with incomes above 200 percent of the federal poverty level, although the effect persisted in both income groups. For both lower- and higher-income adults, the negative effect on perceived health of being uninsured was greater than that of having minority racial or ethnic status. Overall, the extent to which being uninsured negatively affected subjective health (a decrement of 4 points on a 100-point scale) was greater than that of having either of two diseases, cancer or gall bladder disease, and slightly lower than that for arteriosclerosis (Franks et al., 1993b).

Ayanian and colleagues' (2000) analysis of the 1998 BRFSS compared self-

---

[17]A "major decline" in health was defined as a change from excellent, very good, or good health in 1992 to fair or poor health in 1996, or from fair health in 1992 to poor health in 1996 (Baker et al., 2001).

TABLE 3.1 Unadjusted Self-Reported Health Status for 18–64 Year-Old Adults, BRFSS, 1998* (percent)

Health Status	Uninsured ≥ 1 Year	Uninsured <1 Year	Insured All Year
Excellent	18	21	27
Very good	27	32	36
Good	35	33	26
Fair	16	11	8
Poor	4	3	3

*Calculated from Table 1 in Ayanian et al., 2000.
SOURCE: Ayanian et al., 2000.

reported health status among adults 18-64 who were uninsured for a year or longer, those uninsured for less than a year, and those with any kind of insurance, public or private. Table 3.1 presents the unadjusted results for the approximately 163,000 adults surveyed. One in five adults uninsured for a year or longer reported being in fair or poor health, compared with one in seven among those uninsured for less than a year, and one in nine for those with health insurance.

The RAND Health Insurance Experiment

In an experimental study conducted between 1975 and 1982, about 4,000 participants between 14 and 61 years were randomly assigned (in family units) to health insurance plans that differed in the amount of patient cost sharing required, ranging from free care to major deductible plans (95 percent cost sharing, with a maximum of $1,000 per family per year) (Brook et al., 1983; Newhouse et al., 1993). Participants received a lump-sum payment at the beginning of the study to compensate them for their expected out-of-pocket costs if they were in cost-sharing plans. Participants were studied for a three- to five-year period. While persons in plans with any cost sharing had significantly fewer physician visits and hospitalizations than persons in a free-care plan, no difference was found overall between plans with any amount of cost sharing and those with no cost sharing. Free care did result in better outcomes for adults with hypertension, as discussed earlier in this chapter, and in improved visual acuity. This experiment demonstrates both the sensitivity of health care utilization in the general population to cost sharing and the relative insensitivity of short-term (three- to five-year) health outcomes for the general population to cost sharing.

Negative Results

Some studies have reported worse health status for those with health insurance compared to uninsured adults. This result may be attributable to the fact that worse health status may lead to coverage by Medicare or Medicaid, as discussed in Chapter 2 (see Box 2.1) and Chapter 4. However, the competing hypothesis, that health insurance is *not* associated with overall health status, must also be considered.

Hahn and Flood (1995) used NMES to examine health status by both income level and type and duration of insurance coverage. When SES and demographic characteristics, health behaviors, health care utilization, and Social Security disability status were controlled for in the analysis, self-reported health status was seen to be arrayed from highest to lowest as follows:

- privately insured for the full year,
- privately insured for part of the year and uninsured for part of the year,
- uninsured for the full year,
- publicly insured for part of the year, and
- publicly insured for the full year.

The authors concluded that the likeliest explanation for their results was that the poorer health status of those who qualify for public coverage was not fully accounted for in their analytic model, even though qualification on the basis of disability was considered explicitly (Hahn and Flood, 1995). An alternative (and possibly supplementary) hypothesis was that public insurance—Medicaid specifically—provided enrollees with access and services that were less effective than those provided by private insurance. Neither of these possible explanations can be eliminated based on the research that the Committee has reviewed.

A second study by Ross and Mirowsky (2000) based on the Survey of Aging, Status and the Sense of Control (ASOC) examined the claim that being uninsured contributes to the worse health of persons of lower SES. The ASOC survey included 2,600 adults between ages 18 and 95 at baseline in 1995, 38 percent of whom were 60 years or older. Participants were reinterviewed in 1998 (44 percent were lost to follow-up) (Ross and Mirowsky, 2000). Health status, functional status, and chronic conditions reported by participants at baseline were used to predict health status, functional status, and chronic conditions three years later. Changes in these measures between baseline and follow-up were also included as predictors of health status, functional status, and number of chronic conditions at follow-up in 1998. The authors concluded that privately insured and uninsured persons had similar health status at a three-year follow-up, adjusted for baseline health status, chronic conditions, and sociodemo-graphic characteristics, and that publicly insured persons had worse health status than privately insured and uninsured adults (Ross and Mirowsky, 2000).

The Committee does not find this study convincing in its conclusions because of both the study sample and its analytic design. The sample included a large proportion of persons over 65, all of whom have Medicare, and the substantial fraction of participants lost to follow-up differed systematically from those who were reinterviewed. By including *changes* in health condition over the study

BOX 3.12
Specific Committee Findings

• Uninsured adults are less likely than adults with any kind of health coverage to receive preventive and screening services and less likely to receive these services on a timely basis. Health insurance that provides more extensive coverage of preventive and screening services is likely to result in greater and more appropriate use of these services.

• Health insurance may reduce racial and ethnic disparities in the receipt of preventive and screening services.

• Uninsured cancer patients generally have poorer outcomes and are more likely to die prematurely than persons with insurance, largely because of delayed diagnosis. This finding is supported by population-based studies of breast, cervical, colorectal, and prostate cancer and melanoma.

• Uninsured adults with chronic diseases are less likely to receive appropriate care to manage their health conditions than are those who have health insurance. For the five conditions that the Committee examined (diabetes, cardiovascular disease, end-stage renal disease, HIV infection, and mental illness), uninsured patients have worse clinical outcomes than insured patients.

• Uninsured adults with hypertension or high blood cholesterol have diminished access to care, are less likely to be screened, are less likely to take prescription medication if diagnosed, and experience worse health.

• Uninsured persons with diabetes are less likely to receive recommended services. Being without health insurance for longer periods increases the risk of inadequate care for this condition and can lead to uncontrolled blood sugar levels, which, over time, put diabetics at risk for additional chronic disease and disability.

• Uninsured patients with end-stage renal disease begin dialysis with more severe disease than do those who had insurance before beginning dialysis.

period as independent variables along with health measures at baseline, the authors may have built their findings into the predictive model itself. In addition, Medicare beneficiaries with supplemental health insurance were classified as privately insured; thus, those who counted as publicly insured included only those Medicare beneficiaries without supplemental policies (a lower-income subset of all Medicare beneficiaries) and Medicaid beneficiaries. This atypical classification scheme distorts the comparison between those with public and private health insurance.

CONCLUSION

This chapter has presented studies examining the impact of health insurance status on general measures of population health, on health care and clinical outcomes for specific conditions, and on the appropriate use of preventive services for the nonelderly adult population in the United States. This body of research yields

- Uninsured adults with HIV infection are less likely to receive highly effective medications that have been shown to improve survival and die sooner as a result.
- Adults with health insurance that covers any mental health treatment are more likely to receive mental health services and care consistent with clinical practice guidelines than are those without any health insurance or insurance that does not cover mental health conditions.
- Uninsured patients who are hospitalized for a range of conditions experience higher rates of death in the hospital, are likely to receive fewer services, and are more likely to experience substandard care and resultant injury than are insured patients.
- Uninsured persons with traumatic injuries are less likely to be admitted to the hospital, likely to receive fewer services when admitted, and are more likely to die than insured trauma victims.
- Uninsured patients with acute cardiovascular disease are less likely to be admitted to a hospital that performs angiography or revascularization procedures, are less likely to receive these diagnostic and treatment procedures, and are more likely to die in the short term.
- Health insurance reduces the disparity in receipt of services for cardiovascular disease by members of racial and ethnic minority groups.
- Longitudinal population-based studies of the mortality of uninsured and privately insured adults reveal a higher risk of dying prematurely for those who were uninsured at the beginning of the study than for those who initially had private coverage.
- Relatively short (one- to four-year) longitudinal studies document relatively greater decreases in general health status measures for uninsured adults and for those who lost insurance coverage during the period studied than for those with continuous coverage.

largely consistent and significant findings about the relationship between health insurance and health-related outcomes. *In summary, uninsured adults receive health care services that are less adequate and appropriate than those received by patients who have either public or private health insurance, and they have poorer clinical outcomes and poorer overall health than do adults with private health insurance.* The specific findings discussed throughout this chapter are presented in Box 3.12.

The Committee has assessed the research regarding the effects of health insurance status across a range of health conditions and services affecting adults. In each domain examined—

- preventive care and screening services,
- cancer care and outcomes,
- chronic disease management and patient outcomes,
- acute care services and outcomes for hospitalized adults, and
- overall health status and mortality,

health insurance improved the likelihood of appropriate care and was associated with better health outcomes. Health insurance appears to achieve these positive effects in part through facilitating ongoing care with a regular health care provider and reducing financial barriers to obtaining those services that constitute or contribute to appropriate care, including screening services, prescription drugs, and specialty mental health services.

Chapter 4 specifically addresses the question of the difference that providing health insurance to uninsured individuals and populations would make to their health and health care. The Committee assesses the potential impact of health insurance coverage on those uninsured adults who are most at risk for poor or adverse health-related outcomes, including the chronically ill, adults in late middle age, members of ethnic minorities, and adults in lower-income households. The chapter also reviews the features and characteristics of health insurance that account for its effectiveness in achieving better health outcomes, including both continuity of coverage and scope of benefits.

NOTES

BOX 4.1
Conclusions

The Committee's conclusions are supported by the evidence and findings presented in Chapter 3, which are largely based on observational studies.

• Health insurance is associated with better health outcomes for adults and with their receipt of appropriate care across a range of preventive, chronic, and acute care services. Adults without health insurance coverage die sooner and experience greater declines in health status over time than do adults with continuous coverage.

• Adults with chronic conditions, and those in late middle age, are the most likely to realize improved health outcomes as a result of gaining health insurance coverage because of their high probability of needing health care services.

• Population groups that are most at risk of lacking stable health insurance coverage and that have worse health status, including racial and ethnic minorities and lower-income adults, particularly would benefit from increased health insurance coverage. Increased coverage would likely reduce some of the racial and ethnic disparities in the utilization of appropriate health care services and might also reduce disparities in morbidity and mortality among ethnic groups.

• When health insurance affords access to providers and includes preventive and screening services, outpatient prescription drugs, and specialty mental health care, it is more likely to facilitate the receipt of appropriate care than when insurance does not have these features.

• Broad-based health insurance strategies across the entire uninsured population would be more likely to produce the benefits of enhanced health and life expectancy than would "rescue" programs aimed only at the seriously ill.

4

The Difference Coverage Could Make to the Health of Uninsured Adults

Health insurance contributes independently and positively to the health of adults and to the receipt of appropriate preventive services and care for chronic and acute conditions. This overarching conclusion of the Committee rests on the review and synthesis of research evidence presented in Chapter 3. These conclusions take into account the methodological limitations of the largely observational research that supports them, as discussed below.

This final chapter considers the broader implications of the Committee's findings, including an assessment of the health-related benefits of insuring American adults who now lack health insurance coverage. What impact would health insurance coverage have? Relating these findings to the U.S. uninsured population as a whole depends on the characteristics of uninsured Americans, as well as assumptions about the extent to which health insurance would improve the health of those who lack coverage. Projecting or estimating the potential impacts of health insurance on those who lack coverage also entails identifying the features and mechanisms of health insurance promoting the receipt of care that effectively improves health outcomes. This projection, or "what-if" exercise, requires a number of assumptions and careful linking of a sequence of inferences.

As detailed in *Coverage Matters: Insurance and Health Care* (IOM, 2001a), the 30 million American adults without health insurance are disproportionately young, nonwhite, and members of lower-income families. About half of all uninsured adults are between the ages of 18 and 35, a relatively healthy time of life.[1] The

---

[1] Although youth is not itself a risk factor for unmet health care needs, within every band of the age spectrum some of those without health insurance are especially vulnerable. Among young adults, those with special health needs who had coverage as dependents of their parents or through public programs as disabled children and lost it upon reaching age 19, 20, or 21 are at greater risk of having unmet health care needs (Fishman, 2001).

other half are between 35 and 65 years of age. Although older adults are not especially likely to be uninsured, being uninsured is especially risky for older adults because of the much higher incidence of chronic and other illnesses in late middle age.[2] Approximately half of uninsured adults are non-Hispanic whites, more than a quarter are Hispanic, one out of six are African American, and one out of twenty are Asian American (IOM, 2001a). Almost two-thirds of uninsured adults have just 12 years of schooling or less (IOM, 2001a), and half have family incomes under 200 percent of the federal poverty level (Fronstin, 2001b). Most uninsured adults (85 percent) either work or live in families where someone works at least part time (Hoffman and Pohl, 2002).

The causal link between health insurance coverage and better health outcomes cannot be established conclusively by observational studies alone. The studies reviewed in Chapter 3 that compare the health outcomes of insured and uninsured populations, even with the extensive analytical adjustments that make these comparisons more valid, do not answer definitively the question of whether health insurance itself improves health outcomes. Nonetheless, the Committee developed its conclusions based on the substantial consistency of results among the methodologically strongest observational studies and the coherence of these results with the behavioral research evidence that informs the Committee's conceptual model of the mechanisms by which health insurance affects health outcomes (see Figure 1.1).

In order to understand the implications of the research evidence presented here for the population of uninsured Americans, the Committee first considers the findings of the previous chapter as they relate to specific groups within the overall population of uninsured adults. Second, this chapter reviews the features of health insurance plans that research indicates make a difference in health-related outcomes for adults, information that is essential for designing effective policies to extend insurance coverage. Last, the Committee considers the potential benefits that could be achieved by providing health insurance coverage to uninsured adults.

ADULTS MOST AT RISK OF POOR HEALTH

Chronically Ill Adults and the Risk Associated With Aging

Adults who have chronic illnesses face functional limitations and premature death, consequences that might be ameliorated by appropriate health care. Chronic illness and advancing age interact to increase vulnerability to the health effects of being uninsured.

The prevalence of activity-limiting chronic conditions for the population

---

[2]Adults between ages 55 and 65 have an uninsured rate of 14 percent, somewhat below the overall average (17.6 percent) and just half the rate for adults between ages 18 and 25 (Fronstin, 2001b).

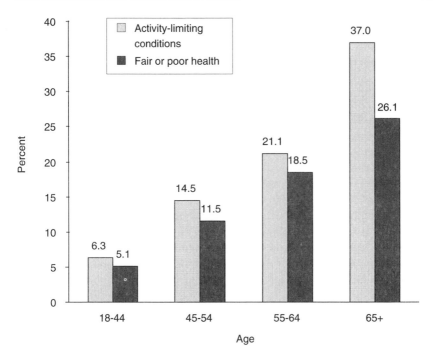

FIGURE 4.1 U.S. population with activity-limiting chronic conditions (1998) and fair or poor health (1999).
SOURCE: NCHS, 2001, Tables 57 and 58.

under age 45 is relatively low and stable, at about 6 percent (NCHS, 2001).[3] Between ages 45 and 55, however, the rate of activity-limiting conditions more than doubles, to 14.5 percent of the population, and it increases to 21 percent for those between ages 55 and 65. For those ages 65 and older, more than one-third (37 percent) have activity limitations due to chronic conditions (Figure 4.1). Likewise, the proportion of the population reporting fair or poor health increases from 5 percent for those between ages 18 and 45 to 11.5 percent for those ages 45–54 and to 18.5 percent for those ages 55–64 (NCHS, 2001). Fully one-quarter of persons 65 and older report being in fair or poor health.

The appropriate use of health care services in screening, early diagnosis, and disease management can reduce the burdens of disability and death due to chronic

---

[3]In the National Health Interview Survey, from which these data are reported, limitations of activity refer to long-term reductions in the capacity to perform activities typical for persons in the same age group as the respondent that are due to a chronic health condition. Such activities include personal care (bathing, dressing, eating), walking, and remembering (NCHS, 2001).

diseases such as cardiovascular disease, cancer, diabetes, depression, HIV infection, kidney disease, and arthritis. Chronically ill persons without health insurance are much less likely than those who are insured to have had a physician visit within a year's time (odds ratio [OR] = 0.5 in Hafner-Eaton, 1993; see also Fish-Parcham, 2001).

Except for those with end-stage renal disease (93 percent of whom have Medicare coverage), chronically ill adults under age 65 are about as likely to be uninsured as are their healthier counterparts. Medicare or Medicaid coverage for disabled adults who reside in the community (i.e., are not in health care institutions) extend to only some of those with chronic conditions. For persons under age 65, 3 million of the 21 million persons under age 65 diagnosed with heart disease, 2 million of the 14 million diagnosed with hypertension, and 1 million of the 8 million diagnosed with arthritis lack health insurance (estimates based on the 1996 Medical Expenditure Panel Survey [MEPS]) (Fish-Parcham, 2001).[4] Fully one-quarter of lower-income (i.e., with family incomes less than 200 percent of the federal poverty level) persons with heart disease, hypertension, or arthritis lacked coverage (Fish-Parcham, 2001).

As the U.S. population ages, both the numbers and the proportion of adults at greater risk of developing health problems are increasing. While the 37.3 million adults in the 55–64 age cohort now represent 8.7 percent of the U.S. population, this age group is projected to grow 2.5 percent each year through 2015—to 61.9 million or almost 20 percent of the total population (Kinsella and Velkoff, 2001). Sixty percent of those workers between ages 55 and 65 who are uninsured, 1.3 million people, report having health problems, and one out of every five adults in this age group, 4.8 million people, has at least one activity limitation due to a chronic condition (Monheit et al., 2001; NCHS, 2001). More than 900,000 adults ages 55–64 in fair or poor health were uninsured in 1999 (Swartz and Stevenson, 2001). Uninsured older adults are much less likely than their insured counterparts to have a regular source of care or to receive cancer or heart disease screenings, as illustrated in Table 4.1 (Powell-Griner et al., 1999).

Older workers and their spouses who have health insurance coverage through the workplace are increasingly at risk of loss of health insurance if they retire before age 65, because employers are increasingly dropping retiree health benefits and raising the costs to retirees of participating in those plans that have survived (GAO, 1998; GAO, 2001a, 2001b; Fronstin and Reno, 2001). Furthermore, while older adults are more likely than young workers to purchase individual insurance policies if they do not have access to workplace coverage, they are also more likely to face higher premiums, benefits exclusions, and refusals of coverage because of their age and health conditions (GAO, 2001a, 2001b; IOM, 2001a; Monheit et al., 2001; Pollitz, 2001). Older women particularly are at risk of not

---

[4]These condition-specific estimates count individuals with multiple conditions more than once.

TABLE 4.1 Adjusted Odds Ratios for Uninsured Versus Insured U.S. Adults Ages 55–64 Years for Selected Characteristics, 1993–1996

Characteristics	Adjusted Odds Ratio[a]	95% Confidence Interval
Health status good, very good, or excellent	0.79	0.68-0.93
Regular source of care	0.25	0.19-0.33
Cost a barrier to care	7.58	6.46-8.91
Last routine checkup ≤2 years	0.25	0.21-0.28
Last Pap test ≤3 years	0.38	0.31-0.46
Last mammogram ≤3 years	0.27	0.23-0.32
Last clinical breast exam ≤2 years	0.32	0.26-0.39
Last blood pressure check ≤ 2 years	0.21	0.16-0.29
Last cholesterol check ≤ 5 years	0.35	0.28-0.43

[a]Adjusted for sex, race, educational level, and marital status.
SOURCE: Adapted from Powell-Griner et al., 1999, Table 3.

having health insurance coverage, because of gender-related employment patterns and a greater likelihood of obtaining coverage as a dependent of an older spouse, who may lose access to spousal workplace coverage upon retirement (Meyer and Pavalko, 1996). For working women, ages 55–64 in good, fair, or poor health, 23 percent lack health insurance, compared with 10 percent of those in excellent or very good health (Monheit et al., 2001). In contrast, health insurance coverage rates for working men in this age group do not vary by health status (Monheit et al., 2001).

Adults with Severe Mental Illnesses

Among chronically ill adults, those with a severe mental illness deserve special attention when considering health insurance coverage because the issues of appropriate care and maintaining coverage are closely related for them.[5] Almost 4.5 million Americans, 2.8 percent of adults over age 18, have a severe mental illness (Narrow et al., 2000). Persons with severe mental illness are more likely to have

---

[5]Severe mental illnesses include schizophrenia, other psychoses, manic-depression (bipolar disorder), and severe forms of other disorders such as major depression (Narrow et al., 2000).

alcohol and substance use disorders than are members of the general population (U.S. Surgeon General, 1999; Narrow et al., 2000).

Persons with chronic mental conditions that include behavioral and psychotic symptoms, who reside outside institutions (including the homeless), may have difficulty meeting the demands of daily living, especially functions such as maintaining employment or health insurance (Pollack and Kronebusch, 2001). Although many persons with severe mental illnesses qualify for Medicare or Medicaid as disabled, their condition may make it difficult for them to maintain continuous coverage through Medicaid, which requires periodic requalification (Bazelon/Milbank, 2000). An estimated 45 percent of persons with a severe mental illness have public insurance. However, even with this relatively high rate of public insurance coverage, 20 percent of adults with a severe mental illness remain uninsured (McAlpine and Mechanic, 2000).

Despite having a serious and chronic condition, only 40–60 percent of persons with a severe mental illness receive any outpatient treatment within a given year (McAlpine and Mechanic, 2000; Narrow et al., 2000). Lacking health insurance is the most commonly reported barrier to receiving care for persons with mental illness (Druss and Rosenheck, 1998). In addition, persons with severe mental illness face exceptional difficulties in obtaining health care apart from mental health services and are more likely to die prematurely from physical conditions than are persons without mental diagnoses (Druss et al., 2001; Jeste and Unuetzer, 2001).

Persons of Lower Socioeconomic Status and Members of Racial and Ethnic Minorities

Adults with lower educational attainment and lower incomes use fewer health services and have worse health outcomes than do better-educated and higher-income adults, and they are also more likely to be uninsured (Preston and Elo, 1995; IOM, 2001a; Shi, 2001).[6] Lower-income persons tend to be uninsured for longer periods than higher-income persons, which increases their risk of poorer health-related outcomes, as discussed in the previous chapter (McBride, 1997; IOM, 2001a). Adults in lower-income families are also substantially more likely to have experienced recent gaps in health insurance coverage as well as being more likely to be uninsured at a given point in time, as illustrated in Figure 4.2 (Hoffman et al., 2001).

African Americans and Hispanics face greater barriers to health care and poorer health outcomes than do non-Hispanic whites and are more likely to lack health insurance, with two and three times the uninsured rate, respectively, of non-Hispanic whites (IOM, 2001a). Among the uninsured who are in families

---

[6]Lower income is defined as having a family income below 200 percent of the federal poverty level or $34,100 for a family of four in 2000.

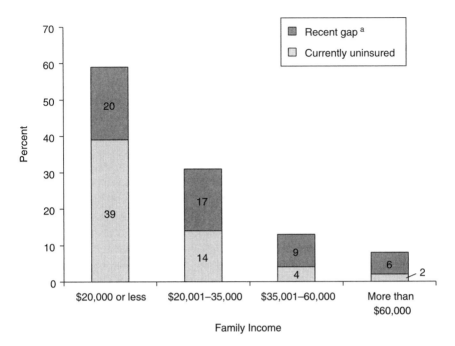

FIGURE 4.2 Percentage of adults in working families who were uninsured within the past two years, by income. [a]Person was insured at the time of the survey but had a period in the past two years without coverage.
SOURCE: Hoffman et al., 2001, Figure 1. Based on the Kaiser/Commonwealth 1997 National Survey of Health Insurance.

with incomes below the federal poverty level (about $17,000 for a family of four in 2000), about 40 percent are members of racial and ethnic minority groups (Mills, 2001). The lack of health insurance thus converges with other risk factors (low socioeconomic status [SES] and minority status) to reduce the likelihood of receiving needed care (IOM, 2001a; Shi, 2001). Although lack of health insurance is only one of several factors that contribute to socioeconomic and ethnic disparities in health, it is an important component and is one of the most amenable to intervention. Health insurance more strongly and consistently influences health care utilization than it does health status. While health insurance may alleviate financial barriers to care and improve the choice of providers, it does not address other individual and societal determinants of poor health and disparate care that are experienced by ethnic minorities and the economically disadvantaged. These include low literacy skills that may interfere with the ability to understand instructions or participate in medical decisions, health beliefs, life-style practices, and environmental influences (Haas and Adler, 2001). In addition, health care providers are not uniformly competent in cross-cultural communication, and this, along with a history of overt racial discrimination, may result in less effective provider–patient interactions (Haas and Adler, 2001; IOM, 2002). Thus, although health insurance by itself will not eliminate ethnic and socioeconomic disparities in health, it may reduce such disparities and improve health-related outcomes for minority and economically disadvantaged groups.

Multiple Jeopardy

The health risks of being uninsured are not randomly distributed throughout the U.S. population, nor are they randomly distributed among the population of uninsured adults. Many of the uninsured belong to one or more of the higher-risk groups just discussed. For these individuals, lacking health insurance represents a more immediate threat to their health and personal well being (Shi, 2001).

The greater risks of poor health for adults in late middle age, those of lower SES, and members of racial and ethnic minority groups make health insurance even more important for these multiply disadvantaged groups because coverage and health services can make more of a positive difference. A corollary of this is that studies of the impact of health care on health outcomes that are based on broader populations may not fully reflect its significant impact on particular subpopulations at heightened risk of poor health outcomes. When these subpopulations are examined separately however, the impact of health care and coverage becomes apparent.

For example, the RAND Health Insurance Experiment demonstrated that persons with lower incomes and worse health status are most affected by cost-sharing requirements. Lower-income adults with hypertension who faced no cost sharing had better blood pressure control than those in plans with any amount of cost sharing. In contrast, overall, the experiment did not find differences in most health outcomes related to cost sharing (Brook et al., 1983; Keeler et al., 1985; Newhouse et al., 1993). Similarly, in a small "natural experiment" among low-income adults in California, the loss of Medi-Cal coverage was accompanied by diminished overall health status and, for those with hypertension, by markedly poorer blood pressure control after six months and one year (Lurie et al., 1984, 1986).[7] Although these larger effects of health insurance on vulnerable populations are diluted in broader, population-based studies, they are present in the results of the research presented in Chapter 3.

FEATURES OF HEALTH INSURANCE THAT IMPROVE HEALTH-RELATED OUTCOMES

Health insurance has different effects depending on the kind and conditions of coverage. With the exception of the RAND Health Insurance Experiment, the

---

[7]Both of these studies are discussed more fully in Chapter 3.

literature review excluded studies that examined patterns of health care use and outcomes only among insured populations. Thus, for example, the Committee's findings do not include comparisons between fee-for-service and managed care plans. Although scope of benefits was not the primary focus of this review, studies of several chronic conditions and utilization of screening services suggest that the magnitude of the health insurance effect is related to the benefits covered. Furthermore, some of the differences reported among those covered by Medicaid, Medicare, and private health insurance can be attributed to differences in the scopes of benefits under these alternative forms of coverage.

Regular Source of Care and Continuity of Coverage

A continuing relationship with a primary provider or system of care is a hallmark of quality health care (IOM, 2001b). Health insurance is effective in improving receipt of appropriate health care in part because it increases access to a regular source of care. Many of the studies reviewed in the previous chapter, particularly in the management of chronic disease and preventive care, confirmed that more appropriate utilization and better outcomes for insured adults could be accounted for by the greater likelihood of having a regular source of care compared to uninsured adults and those with a recent gap in coverage. Stable health insurance coverage maintains access to a regular source of care over time.

Having health insurance coverage that does not afford access to a regular source of care for any reason (e.g., geographical scarcity, restricted provider pools, inadequate provider participation) may result in outcomes for insured adults that differ little from those for uninsured adults. Having health insurance with frequent breaks in coverage that disrupt access to a regular source of care is also less effective in improving health-related outcomes than is continuous coverage (Lurie et al., 1986; Burstin et al., 1998; Hoffman et al., 2001). In particular, Medicaid enrollees may have inadequate access to a regular source of care both because of insufficient provider participation and because enrollment in Medicaid tends to be sporadic, as discussed below.

The performance of health insurance plans and programs in facilitating a regular and continuing care relationship for enrollees should be a key factor in the design of any health insurance coverage reform.

Scope of Benefits

The scope of health insurance benefits also influences how coverage affects health-related outcomes. As noted in Chapter 1, there is no standard or calibrated "dose" of health insurance across the studies that examine health insurance effects. Private health insurance plans vary widely in terms of their benefits, cost-sharing provisions, and conditions by which providers participate in them (IOM, 2001a). They may or may not cover preventive services, prescription drugs, or specialty mental health services; impose substantial deductible or coinsurance requirements;

restrict access to specialists; or require each enrollee to have a primary care provider.

Coverage of preventive services, prescription drugs, and mental health services varies considerably among health insurance plans. These services, however, are critical elements of appropriate health care that can improve outcomes for conditions such as cancer, cardiovascular disease, diabetes, HIV infection, and depression. Chronically ill adults whose conditions require pharmaceutical therapies are more likely to follow their treatment regimens if they have insurance coverage for prescription drugs (Huttin et al., 2000).

The distinctive benefit packages of public health insurance programs affect the outcomes that have been reviewed here. For example, the superior results for Medicaid and Medicare enrollees with respect to mental health care may be attributed to the more extensive coverage of these services than that available under many private insurance plans. Also, the coverage of preventive services and prescription drugs by Medicaid may account for the more appropriate receipt of screenings and chronic disease care, comparable to that for those enrolled in private health plans, by those enrolled in Medicaid.

Ease of access to providers is another aspect of plan benefits that affects the impact of health insurance coverage on outcomes. These considerations apply to both public and private insurance programs and plans. Access may be administratively restricted (e.g., with appointment protocols) or enhanced (e.g., with assignment of a specific primary care provider) within managed care plans. Payment rates and arrangements also affect the willingness of providers to participate and, consequently, affect the access of enrollees to care. Adequate access to providers, under both managed care and fee-for-service programs, is particularly problematic within some Medicaid programs, as discussed in the following section.

The Special Case of Medicaid

As evident in several individual study results for overall health status, cancer outcomes, and hospital-based care, adults with Medicaid coverage frequently fare no better and sometimes fare worse than uninsured patients in their health-related outcomes, even when observations are adjusted for demographic factors and health status at the beginning of the study period. Two factors contribute to the distinctive outcomes for Medicaid enrollees: the structure and operation of Medicaid as an insurance program and the characteristics of the population that qualifies for Medicaid coverage.

The programmatic features of Medicaid that contribute to worse health-related outcomes among its enrollees include provider participation and payment levels and limited coverage periods. Low provider payment rates, in both the fee-for-service and the capitated sectors, reduce access to health care services for Medicaid enrollees in many states and localities (IOM, 2000a). (Medicaid payment levels and conditions of provider participation vary among states, as do health sector services and resources more generally.) Medicaid enrollees often find themselves limited to much the same set of overtaxed safety-net providers as uninsured adults, with concomitant delays in getting appointments and referrals to specialists and little continuity of care (IOM, 2000a). Medicaid's limited coverage periods also weaken any positive effects of insurance. Medicaid coverage tends to be intermittent, with adults gaining or losing coverage as their income, employment, or health status changes (McBride, 1997; Davidoff et al., 2001). In one recent study based on the federal Survey of Income and Program Participation, the median length of time that adults under age 65 maintained Medicaid enrollment was just five months (Tin and Castro, 2001). In some states, Medicaid requires eligibility redeterminations as frequently as monthly, and some people lose coverage simply because they did not meet administrative requirements. As a consequence of the intermittency of Medicaid coverage, adults identified as covered by Medicaid at one point in time may not achieve the benefits that continuous health insurance coverage can provide.

The second aspect that contributes to the worse outcomes of Medicaid enrollees—its distinctive eligibility criteria—is discussed in Chapter 2 (see Box 2.1). Adults who are eligible for Medicaid are low income and often are either disabled or incur significant health care expenses. Each of these factors is associated with relatively poor health status. Furthermore, among all adults who are eligible for Medicaid coverage, those who actually enroll in the program are likely to be those who have already had encounters with the health care system (Davidoff et al., 2001). This operational feature of Medicaid can distort the results of studies of insurance status and outcomes. For example, a Medicaid enrollee being treated for breast cancer may have developed the disease long before enrolling in Medicaid, yet her late-stage cancer diagnosis, a worse outcome, is attributed to the publicly insured (rather than uninsured) group if cancer registry or hospital records identify her as covered by Medicaid at the time of diagnosis (Perkins et al., 2001).

Medicaid coverage is not worse than no coverage at all, as a facile review of study results might suggest. Medicaid is a program with structural features that limit its ability to deliver to enrollees all of the potential benefits of health insurance coverage and it serves adult populations with multiple health risks.

INSURING THE UNINSURED: IMPROVING HEALTH OUTCOMES

How would health care utilization and health outcomes be affected by providing adults who now lack coverage with health insurance? What can we learn from the largely observational body of research on the impact of health insurance on utilization and outcomes about the impacts of providing those Americans who are most at risk of lacking health insurance with such coverage? First, we can expect that upon gaining coverage, uninsured adults would

- use more health care services,
- receive more appropriate preventive care, and
- better manage their chronic conditions.

Health insurance would improve the chances that currently uninsured adults would have a regular source of care. Providers would be more likely to provide appropriate services to a patient with a condition of given severity if that patient had health insurance, but could also be more likely to provide services that were not clearly clinically indicated.[8] **Most importantly, if adults who now lack health insurance were to be insured on a stable and ongoing basis, their health status would likely be better than it would be without health insurance, and their risk of dying prematurely would be reduced.**

The Committee recognizes that health insurance alone will not eliminate disparities in access to health care among the population now without health insurance nor will it equalize health outcomes among socioeconomically diverse groups. Such disparities persist in countries such as Great Britain and Canada that do have universal health insurance programs (Marmot et al., 1991; Hamilton et al., 1997; Ho et al., 2000). See Boxes 2.2 and 2.3 for further discussion of disparities related to race and ethnicity and SES. Nevertheless, health insurance is associated with better physical functioning, health status, and health-related quality of life (Baker et al., 2001; Franks et al., 1993b; Cunningham et al., 1995; Penson et al., 2001). Health insurance is also associated with better survival, both overall and for adults with specific conditions such as cancer, cardiovascular diseases, and HIV infection. Appendix D presents estimates for the U.S. population as a whole of the differential mortality risks for adults with and without health insurance, as illustrative of the potential reductions in mortality among uninsured adults that could follow from insuring the entire U.S. population.

However, the survival benefits of having health insurance coverage can be achieved fully only when health insurance is acquired well before the development of advanced disease. The problem of later diagnosis and higher mortality among uninsured women with breast cancer, for example, cannot be solved by insuring women once their disease is diagnosed. Greater use of preventive services, early detection of disease, and effective, continuous management of health conditions account for many of the benefits that health insurance provides its enrollees. A patient with an ongoing relationship with a health care provider is more likely to receive appropriate medical attention and services early in the development of an illness or disease process rather than only once the condition

---

[8]This conclusion is supported by the findings in Chapter 3, particularly those for hospital-based care (including cardiovascular disease and trauma treatments). See also, "Physician Response to Patient Insurance Status in Ambulatory Care Clinical Decision-Making" (Mort et al., 1996) for primary care physicians' responses to hypothetical clinical scenarios that included information about the patient's insurance status.

has become acute or difficult to treat. Insurance coverage can facilitate such a relationship and provide the financial means for patients and their provider of first contact to obtain beneficial health care services. **The Committee concludes that broad-based health insurance strategies across the entire uninsured population would be more likely to produce the benefits of enhanced health and life expectancy than would "rescue" programs aimed only at the seriously ill.**

Finally, the evidence presented in this report accounts for only some of the benefits and advantages that health insurance provides. The Committee's first report, *Coverage Matters,* identified financial risk reduction and economic security as major benefits of health insurance that accrued to everyone with coverage, whether or not they happened to use it. These considerations will be examined again from the standpoint of family well being in the Committee's next report.

This research review did not examine patient satisfaction or quantify the sense of being valued when professional and caring attention is provided in painful, stressful, or frightening circumstances. Yet these less tangible qualities are just as real as improvements in survival rates. Furthermore, they are more likely to be achieved in health care settings and healing relationships in which people may confidently make a claim on health care providers' time and resources. Adults without health insurance are less likely to feel entitled to a provider's attention when they seek care and indeed, uninsured adults are less likely to seek needed care than are those with health insurance (Kaiser Commission, 2000).[9]

Thus, although this report has focused almost entirely on health-related outcomes, the most quantifiable and extensively measured personal consequences of health insurance, they account for only some of the benefits of coverage. Financial security and stability, peace of mind, alleviation of pain and suffering, improved physical function, disabilities avoided or delayed, and gains in life expectancy constitute an array of benefits that accrue to members of our society who have health insurance. For many of the 40 million uninsured Americans, these benefits remain out of reach.

---

[9]See Ferrer (2001), for an account of the circumstances under which uninsured persons obtain care in overtaxed safety-net facilities that supports these points.

A

A Conceptual Framework for Evaluating the Consequences of Uninsurance: A Cascade of Effects

The Committee's general conceptual framework for evaluating the consequences of uninsurance is depicted in Figure A.1. This overall conceptualization was the basis of the Committee's model for this report on health outcomes, as depicted in Figure 1.1. Both versions of the conceptual framework are based upon a widely employed behavioral model of access to health services that explicates the processes of health care and health-related outcomes for individuals (Andersen and Davidson, 2001).

Figure A.1 groups variables into the categories of *resources* that promote or enable one to obtain health care; personal or community *characteristics* that favor or predispose action to obtain health care; and *needs* for health care, as articulated by those in need, determined by health care providers, or identified by researchers and decision makers. Judgments about how susceptible a variable is to change are implicit in the categories of resources, characteristics, and needs. Resources are considered, at least theoretically, as more open to change. Characteristics are less manipulable and needs comprise a heterogeneous grouping, with some needs more changeable than others.

The overall model begins with the primarily economic determinants of health insurance status in Panel 1 of the figure. Panel 2 displays, in compressed form, the resources, characteristics, and needs of both individuals and communities that affect the process of obtaining access to health care. Panel 3 displays the consequences of uninsurance that are being examined in the Committee's various reports. These effects cascade from the smallest unit of analysis, the individual, to increasingly larger units, first that of the family and then the community. Panel 2 and one element of Panel 3, "Health Outcomes for Individuals," represent the focus of *Care Without Coverage*. These sections of the overall framework are expanded upon in Figure 1.1.

The arrows and arrangement of the boxes in Figure A.1 indicate hypothesized causal and temporal relationships. As reflected by the figure, the relationships among factors that determine health insurance status, access to health care, and health, social, and economic outcomes are dynamic with multiple feedbacks. For example, as discussed earlier in this report, health status is both an outcome variable in this model and an important determinant of health insurance status, the individual and family-level resource that is the independent variable of interest in this report.

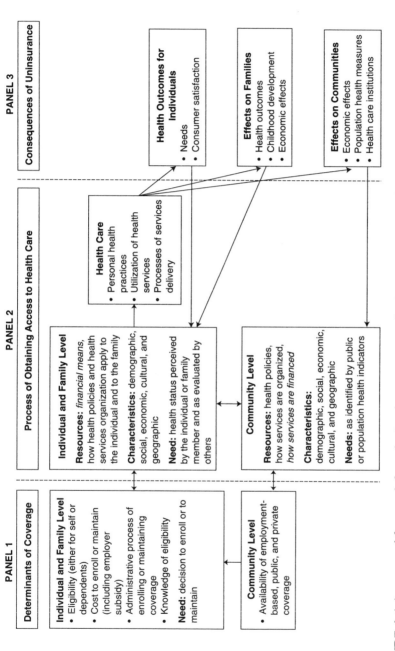

FIGURE A.1 A conceptual framework for evaluating the consequences of uninsurance. NOTE: Italics indicate terms that include direct measures of health insurance coverage. Reprinted from *Coverage Matters: Insurance and Health Care* (IOM, 2001a).

The following text appears within the figure:

PANEL 1

Determinants of Coverage

Individual and Family Level
- Eligibility (either for self or dependents)
- Cost to enroll or maintain (including employer subsidy)
- Administrative process of enrolling or maintaining coverage
- Knowledge of eligibility

Need: decision to enroll or to maintain

Community Level
- Availability of employment-based, public, and private coverage

PANEL 2

Process of Obtaining Access to Health Care

Individual and Family Level

Resources: *financial means, how health policies and health services organization apply to the individual and to the family*

Characteristics: demographic, social, economic, cultural, and geographic

Need: health status perceived by the individual or family member and as evaluated by others

Community Level

Resources: health policies, how services are organized, *how services are financed*

Characteristics: demographic, social, economic, cultural, and geographic

Needs: as identified by public or population health indicators

Health Care
- Personal health practices
- Utilization of health services
- Processes of services delivery

PANEL 3

Consequences of Uninsurance

Health Outcomes for Individuals
- *Needs*
- Consumer satisfaction

Effects on Families
- Health outcomes
- Childhood development
- Economic effects

Effects on Communities
- Economic effects
- Population health measures
- Health care institutions

B

Primary Research Literature Review

Sample Size/Data Source

Overall Health Status/Mortality

Baker et al. (2001)
Lack of Health Insurance and Decline
in Overall Health in Late Middle Age.
N Engl J Med

7,577 participants in Health & Retirement
Survey. 51-61 yrs at baseline in 1992; 1994;
1996

Brook et al. (1983)
Does Free Care Improve Adults' Health?
Results from a Randomized Controlled
Trial. *N Engl J Med*

3,958 participants ages 14-61 yrs at 6 sites.
1975-1982

Franks et al. (1993a)
Health Insurance and Mortality.
Evidence From a National Cohort. *JAMA*

4,694 adults ≥25, UI or privately insured at
baseline NHANES I,Epi. Followup Study,
1971-1987

Franks et al. (1993b)
Health Insurance and Subjective Health
Status: Data from the 1987 National
Medical Expenditure Survey. *Am J
Pub Health*

12,036 adults ages 25-64, 1987 NMES

Hahn and Flood. (1995)
No Insurance, Public Insurance, and
Private Insurance: Do These Options
Contribute to Differences in General
Health? *J Health Care Poor Underserved*

36,259 adults 18-64. 1987 NMES

Kasper et al. (2000)
Gaining and Losing Health Insurance:
Strengthening the Evidence for Effects on
Access to Care and Health Outcomes.
Med Care Res Rev

1,400 families with at least 1 member <65;
3,142 persons, Kaiser Survey of Family Heath
Experience, 1995–1997

Outcome Measures	Findings

Major decline in health
between 1992 and 1996

21.6% of continuously UI, 16.1% of intermittently UI, 8.3% of continuously insured had a major health decline over 4-yr period. Continuously UI had an adjusted relative risk of 1.6 compared to continuously insured of a major health decline and an RR of 1.2 to develop a mobility limitation. For the intermittently insured, these respective RRs were 1.4 and 1.2

M.D. visits; hospitalization
mortality; clinical measures;
overall heath status

Over a 3-5 year period, participants were randomly assigned to HI plans with different cost sharing, from free care to major deductible. No difference was found, overall, on 8 of 10 measures of health status and health habits between cost-sharing and free-care groups. For low-income persons with high BP, diastolic BP was lower by 3 mm Hg in free-care group. Free care resulted in improved vision overall

Mortality

Over a 13-17 year follow-up period, the mortality hazard ratio was 1.25 for uninsured adults $\geq$25 years as compared with privately insured adults at baseline (CI: 100-1.55). Adjusted for health status and health behaviors as well as for demographics and SES. No interaction effects found

Multiple health status
measures

Lacking insurance is associated with lower subjective health status, relative to privately insured, independent of other risk factors. This relationship was found in those at both higher and lower income levels (above and below 200% FPL). Uninsured had less heart disease, more strokes and rheumatism, worse physical and role function, worse MH status. 11 chronic conditions controlled for

Self-reported health status
stratified by age and income

UI have lower health status than those with private coverage. Health status of adults with public insurance is lowest of all. Authors speculate that poorer health status leads to public coverage and/or public insurance differs from private insurance

Measures of access;
self-reported health status

Loss of insurance reduces access to care 2 years later. Those with Medicaid who lost coverage were more likely than those still covered by Medicaid to report no RSC (35% vs. 12%). Overall, no significant differences in health status after loss of health insurance, except for those losing Medicaid, who initially reported better health, but lost the gains over time

Sample Size/Data Source

Lurie et al. (1984)
Termination from Medi-Cal: Does It
Affect Health? *New Engl J Med*

Lurie et al. (1986)
Termination of Medi-Cal Benefits:
A Followup Study One Year Later
New Engl J Med

215 medically indigent adult patients at
UCLA Ambulatory Care Center and comparison
group of 109 patients whose benefits were
not terminated

Ross and Mirowsky (2000)
Does Medical Insurance Contribute to
Socioeconomic Differentials in Health?
Milbank Q

2,592 adults 18–95 yrs at baseline in 1995;
1,452 at follow-up in 1998. Survey of Aging,
Status, and the Sense of Control

Short and Lair (1994-1995)
Health Insurance and Health Status:
Implications for Financing Health Care
Reform. *Inquiry*

7,750 children ages 1–18; 17,341 adults 18-64;
1987 NMES

Sorlie et al. (1994)
Mortality in the Uninsured Compared
with That in Persons with Public and
Private Health Insurance. *Arch Intern Med*

147,779 adults ages 25–64,
Current Population Survey, 1982–1986

Preventive Services

Ayanian et al. (2000)
Unmet Health Needs of Uninsured
Adults in the United States. *JAMA*

105,764 adults ages 18–64 (1997);
117,364 (1998); long-term UI (9.7%),
short-term UI (4.3%), insured (86.0%); BRFSS

Outcome Measures	Findings

General health status; BP control; patient satisfaction; getting needed care

Two cohorts compared: one poor, chronically ill, and uninsured and one poor, chronically ill, and insured; 50% of the uninsured were able to identify an RSC compared to 96% (94% in 1986) of the insured. In 1984 study, 38% of the uninsured thought they could get care whenever they needed it compared to 93% of the insured. In 1986 study, 39% of the uninsured said they could get care whenever needed vs. 80% of the insured; 68% of the uninsured reported needing but not getting care vs. 17% of the insured. BP control significantly deteriorated for hypertensive uninsured individuals. Impossible to isolate the negative consequences of losing Medicaid from accompanying disruption in continuity of care at UCLA clinics. Satisfaction, access, health status worse after losing Medicaid

Health status; chronic conditions; functional status

Longitudinal study. No difference in chronic conditions between uninsured and privately insured. Those with Medicare and Medicaid report more chronic conditions than uninsured. No difference between UI, Medicaid, and those with private insurance in health status or physical functioning

Self-reported health status; chronic conditions

Examines how health affects HI status. Health of those with public insurance is worse than those with private insurance. Often significantly different from uninsured, who had fewer chronic conditions. Age and other covariates not controlled for

Standardized mortality ratio

With adjustment for age and income, UI in 3 of 4 race–gender strata had higher mortality over 5-year follow-up than those with employer-provided insurance, with RRs of 1.2 for white men, 1.5 for black men, 1.5 for white women, and 0.8 for black women. White uninsured workers had relative mortality risks 1.2 (men) and 1.3 (women) times higher than insured workers. Not adjusted for baseline health

Access to physician; access to preventive care; self-reported health status

Long-term UI ($\geq$1 year) adults were much more likely than short-term (<1 year) UI and insured adults not to have had a routine check-up in the last two years (42.8%, 22.3%, and 17.8%, respectively). Deficits in cancer screening, cardiovascular risk reduction, and diabetes were more pronounced among long-term UI adults than among insured adults

Sample Size/Data Source

Burstin et al. (1998)
The Effect of Change of Health
Insurance on Access to Care. *Inquiry*

2,315 patients who presented to EDs at 5
urban teaching hospitals in Boston, 1993

Cetjin et al. (1999)
Adherence to Colposcopy Among
Women with HIV Infection.
J Acquire Immune Defic Syndr

462 women with or at risk for HIV infection,
1994–1995

Faulkner and Schauffler (1997)
The Effect of Health Insurance
Coverage on the Appropriate Use of
Recommended Clinical Preventive
Services. *Am J Prev Med*

53,981 adults ages 18–64; BRFSS, 1991

Powell-Griner et al. (1999)
Health Coverage and Use of Preventive
Services Among the Near Elderly in the
United States. *Am J Pub Health*

449,604 adults ages 55–64; BRFSS, 1993–1996

Solis et al. (1990)
Acculturation, Access to Care, and Use
of Preventive Services by Hispanics:
Findings from HHANES 1982-1984.
Am J Pub Health

Hispanic adults 20–74 yrs; HHANES, 1982–1984

Wagner and Guendelman (2000)
Healthcare Utilization Among Hispanics:
Findings From the 1994 Minority
Health Survey. *Am J Manag Care*

1,001 Hispanic respondents, 1994

Outcome Measures	Findings

Outcome Measures	Findings
Regular physician; physician follow-up; delays in seeking care; preventive care	Those who lost their insurance had a greater likelihood compared with the privately insured of having no regular physician (OR = 2.63), no physician follow-up (OR = 2.03), and delays in seeking care (OR = 2.21) than those who changed insurance plans (respectively, OR = 0.90, 0.94, and 1.67). Those who lost insurance were less likely to get vaccines (OR=0.24), check-ups in prior year (OR = 0.43), mammograms (OR = 0.61), and stool guaiac testing (OR = 0.68) than those who changed insurance (respectively, ORs = 1.06, 1.32, 0.97, and 1.08)
Colposcopy within 6 months of abnormal cytology finding	HI predicted adherence in multiple logistic regression, but not in bivariate analysis. Sample reflects national population of HIV-positive women
Preventive care; use of preventive services	Higher level of insurance coverage is positively associated with receiving recommended clinical preventive services. Women are more likely than men to receive preventive care. For both men and women, those with no coverage for preventive services are less likely to receive them than those whose health plans cover some or most preventive care (OR = 0.5)
Health status; RSC; cost as barrier to care; Pap test; mammogram; CBE; BP and cholesterol check	Adjusted for sex, race, education, and marital status, UI adults 55-64 less likely than insured to have good or better health (OR = 0.8), RSC (OR = 0.25), more likely to report cost as barrier to care (OR = 7.6), less likely to have check-up (OR = 0.25), Pap test (OR = 0.38), mammogram (OR = 0.27), CBE (OR = 0.32), BP check (OR = 0.2), cholesterol check (OR = 0.35)
Use of preventive services; access to care	Health insurance is independently associated with preventive services even with RSC taken into account. Women were more likely than men to have an RSC. Compared with Cuban Americans and Puerto Ricans, fewer Mexican Americans had any type of health insurance coverage (73.7%, 76.3%, and 66%, respectively)
Use of health services; perception of health status	UI were less likely than those with HI to get any care and used less care (OR = 0.4). Immigrant Hispanics were less likely to use preventive services than U.S.-born Hispanics. Mexican Americans and Puerto Ricans were less likely than other Hispanics to use preventive services (OR = 0.5)

	Sample Size/Data Source
Waidmann and Rajan (2000) Race and Ethnic Disparities in Health Care Access and Utilization: An Examination. *Med Care Res Rev*	Respondents to telephone survey, 1997
Woolhandler and Himmelstein (1988) Reverse Targeting of Preventive Care Due to Lack of Health Insurance. *JAMA*	10,653 women ages 45–64; NHIS, 1982

Screening

Breen et al. (2001) Progress in Cancer Screening Over a Decade. Results of Cancer Screening from the 1987, 1992, and 1998 NHIS. *J Natl Cancer Inst*	Adult respondents; NHIS, 1982, 1987, and 1998
Gordon et al. (1998) Type of Health Coverage and the Likelihood of Being Screened for Cancer. *Med Care*	5,847 interviews; California BRFSS, 1989, 1990
Hsia et al. (2000) The Importance of Health Insurance as a Determinant of Cancer Screening: Evidence from the Women's Health Initiative. *Prev Med*	55,278 women in the Women's Health Initiative Observational Study, 1994–1997
Moran et al. (2000) Factors Influencing Use of the Prostate-Specific Antigen Screening Test in Primary Care. *Am J Manag Care*	4,772 records of male patients ≥ 50; 109 PCPs surveyed, CO 1992–1994
Mosen et al. (1998) Is Access to Medical Care Associated with Receipt of HIV Testing and Counseling? *AIDS Care*	217 patients hospitalized with a HIV-related illness at Los Angeles hospital, 1992–1993

Outcome Measures	Findings
Several measures of access to care and use of health services	HI is associated with differences in use of services and, to a lesser extent, with health status. HI accounts for 33% of the difference between Latinos and non-Hispanic whites (37% of the difference between blacks and whites) in having an RSC, 19% (16%) of the difference in mammography, and 4% (3%)of the difference in health status. The contribution of HI to these racial–ethnic differences varies greatly by region and state
Receipt of preventive health services	UI women 45-64 are less likely to receive BP checks, Pap smears, CBE, or glaucoma exams
Receipt of Pap smear, mammogram, FOBT, sigmoidoscopy	RSC and health insurance are independently and strongly associated with receipt of services. Racial differences (black–white) are greater for UI than for insured. UI were less likely than privately insured to obtain a mammography (OR = 0.5), a Pap smear (OR = 0.37), or colorectal cancer screening (OR = 0.34 for men; 0.63 for women). Those with a RSC were more likely to receive a mammogram (OR = 3.9), a Pap smear (OR = 4.7), or colorectal cancer screening (OR = 5.2 for men; 3.5 for women)
Receipt of Pap smear, mammogram, FOBT, sigmoidoscopy	RSC is best predictor of receiving Pap smear, mammogram, FOBT, sigmoidoscopy, or colorectal screening (OR = 5.2 for men; 3.5 for women). Trends in ORs for UI to private FFS plans suggest lower use by UI, but not statistically significant
Breast, cervical, and olorectal cancer screening	Among women < 65, UI less likely to receive cancer screening, independent of having a RSC. UI less likely than privately insured to have mammogram within 2 years (OR = 0.30); to have Pap smear within 3 years (OR = 0.34); to have sigmoidoscopy or FOBT within 5 years (OR = 0.50). Reference group is private prepaid plan enrollees
Prostate cancer screening: PSA and DRE	Screening for prostate cancer increased significantly between 1992 and 1994. Trend toward greater screening for privately insured vs. UI, but no significant differences
Pre-hospital HIV testing; postdiagnosis receipt of HIV preventive services	Regular source of care has positive effect on receipt of testing and counseling. Health insurance status is not related. Services through VA positively associated with getting preventive counseling. Limited generalizability because of small samples and low response rate

Sample Size/Data Source

Perez and Tsou (1995)
Prostate Cancer Screening Practices:
Differences Between Clinic and Private
Patients. *Mt Sinai J Med*

142 male patients >40 yrs

Potosky et al. (1998)
The Association Between Health Care
Coverage and the Use of Cancer
Screening Tests. *Med Care*

9,455 adults; NHIS, 1992

Cervical and Breast Cancer Screening

Burack et al. (1993)
Patterns of Use of Mammography
Among Inner-City Detroit Women:
Contrasts Between a Health Department,
HMO, and Private Hospital. *Med Care*

2,880 inner-city minority women >40 yrs,
1988–1989

Bush and Langer (1998)
The Effects of Insurance Coverage and
Ethnicity on Mammography Utilization
in a Postmenopausal Population.
West J Med

2,453 postmenopausal women 50–79 yrs;
San Diego, 1993

Cummings et al. (2000)
Predictors of Screenings Mammography:
Implications for Office Practice.
Arch Fam Med

843 women ≥50 yrs in rural communities

Eger and Peipert (1996)
Risk Factors for Noncompliance in a
Colposcopy Clinic. *Journal of
Reproductive Medicine*

200 hospital patients, 1992 data

Evans et al. (1998)
Factors Associated with Repeat
Mammography in a New York State
Public Health Screening Program.
J Public Health Manag Pract

9,485 female participants in a breast cancer
screening outreach program

Outcome Measures	Findings
Prostate cancer screening: PSA and DRE	No difference found between private practice and clinic populations in the frequency of DRE. Private patients were much more likely to receive PSA, 68% compared to 10%
Receipt of Pap smear, mammogram, FOBT, sigmoidoscopy, and DRE	UI less likely than Medicaid and private enrollees to receive preventive services. Mammograms (OR = 0.27), clinical breast exams (OR =0.33), Pap smears (0R = 0.43), fecal occult blood tests (OR = 0.29), or digital rectal exams (OR = 0.28). Medicaid FFS enrollees were more likely to receive a Pap smear than private enrollees (OR = 1.6). UI findings on receipt of sigmoidoscopy not statistically significant. OR comparison group is private managed care
Mammography referral; use of mammography	No differences found by health insurance status. HI status effects vary by site of care. Patient with more visits more likely to have mammography. Study population had access to primary care with frequent utilization
Use of mammography	Mammography use is higher among insured postmenopausal women than their uninsured counterparts with an RSC, but not among insured women without an RSC
Mammography screening; CBE; Pap smear	HI may be an important enabling factor in predicting screening mammography. In bivariate analysis of any HI vs. UI; RR for those with RSC = 1.6; for those without RSC, RR = 1.4. HI is not significant when separate variables for having a Pap smear and receiving a CBE are included in the model
Rate of compliance with colposcopy	Noncompliant women were more likely to be UI or to have Medicaid (OR = 2.4; 95% CI: 0.85–6.7)
Mammography screening	HI not significantly associated with returning for regular mammogram screening in multivariate analysis. Could not account for mammography elsewhere

Sample Size/Data Source

Hayward et al. (1988) Who Gets Screened for Cervical and Breast Cancer? *Arch Intern Med*	4,659 female respondents to a telephone survey, 1986
Jennings-Dozier and Lawrence (2000) Sociodemographic Predictors of Adherence to Annual Cervical Cancer Screening in Minority Women. *Cancer Nurs*	204 minority women
Kirkmann-Liff and Kronenfeld (1992) Access to Cancer Screening Services for Women. *Am J Pub Health*	3,100 women, Arizona, 1989
Mandelblatt et al. (1999) Breast and Cervix Cancer Screening Among Multiethnic Women: Role of Age, Health, and Source of Care. *Prev Med*	1,420 respondents to a telephone survey in New York City, 1992
O'Malley, A., et al. (1997) Continuity of Care and the Use of Breast and Cervical Cancer Screening Services in a Multiethnic Community. *Arch Intern Med*	(Same sample as above)
O'Malley, M., et al. (2001) The Association of Race/Ethnicity, Socioeconomic Status, and Physician Recommendation for Mammography: Who Gets the Message About Breast Cancer Screening? *Am J Pub Health*	2,000 women ≥50 yrs; survey of 10 rural counties, 1993–1994
U.S. Department of Health and Human Services (1998) *Self Reported Use of Mammography and Insurance Status Among Women Aged ≥40 Years—1991–1992 and 1996–1997*	53,188–77,834 women ≥40 yrs BRFFS, 1991–1992, 1996–1997
Zambrana et al. (1999) Use of Cancer Screening Services by Hispanic Women: Analyses by Subgroup. *Prev Med*	2,391 Hispanic women; NHIS, 1990, 1992

Outcome Measures	Findings

Receipt of preventive care; screening | Positive association between health insurance and screening procedures. UI were less likely to have Pap smears (OR = 0.47), breast examinations (OR = 0.36), and mammography (OR = 0.41). Lower income was also a risk factor for not receiving these services

Annual Pap testing | Black women with HI were more likely to receive annual Pap testing than UI black women (OR = 3.8, 95% CI: 0.53–6.85). Hispanic women who received annual Pap testing were more likely to have health insurance (57.5 vs. 42.5%). Reported statistics are not internally consistent

Receipt of Pap smear and mammogram | Low-income UI women significantly less likely than those with either public or private insurance to receive Pap smears (OR = 0.44) and mammograms (OR = 0.29)

Mammogram; Pap smear; CBE; access to care | For Latina and black women in New York City, health insurance is independently important in a multivariable model. For UI, those with RSC are more likely to have had a recent Pap smear (OR = 1.3); more likely to have a recent CBE (OR = 1.5), and more likely to have had a recent mammogram (OR = 2.0). Significant interaction term between insurance and extent of relationship with usual care provider, but coefficient not stated

UI women less likely than insured women to get recommendation for mammogram (OR = 0.63)

Use of mammography | UI women are less likely to receive mammography than insured women (OR = 0.63). Race is not a factor after controlling for SES

Receipt of mammography in previous 2 yrs | Rates of mammography are increasing for both insured and UI, but UI still receive fewer services than insured. For insured women the rates for mammography within the past 2 years increased from 65 to 71%; for UI, from 40 to 46%

Access to health services; regular source of care; cancer screening | Usual source of care is important for all screening services. Health insurance increases mammography use only. UI less likely than privately insured to get mammography (OR = 0.6)

Sample Size/Data Source

Cancer

Ayanian et al. (1993)
The Relation Between Health
Insurance Coverage and Clinical
Outcomes Among Women with Breast
Cancer. *N Engl J Med*

6,026 women 35–64 yrs, NJ State Cancer
Registry, 1985–1987

Berg et al. (1977)
Economic Status and Survival of
Cancer Patients. *Cancer*

Tumor Registry University of Iowa
Hospitals, 1940–1969

Ferrante et al. (2000)
Clinical and Demographic Predictors of
Late-Stage Cervical Cancer.
Arch Fam Med

852 women with invasive cervical cancer;
Florida Cancer Data System, 1994

Gorey et al. (2000)
An International Comparison of Cancer
Survival: Metropolitan Toronto,
Ontario and Honolulu, Hawaii.
Am J Pub Health

7,590 breast and 4,495 prostate cancer cases
in adults ≥25 yrs, 1986–1990

Lee-Feldstein et al. (2000)
The Relationship of HMOs, Health
Insurance, and Delivery Systems to
Breast Cancer Outcomes. *Med Care*

1,788 women <65 diagnosed with breast
cancer; Cancer Surveillance Program, Region 3,
California, 1987-1993

Penson et al. (2001)
The Association Between Socioeconomic
Status, Health Insurance Coverage, and
Quality of Life in Men with Prostate
Cancer. *J Clin Epidemiol*

4,626 patients from 25 communities
CaPSURE database 1995–1998

Perkins et al. (2001)
Breast Cancer Stage at Diagnosis in
Relation to Duration of Medicaid
Enrollment. *Med Care*

10,016 women 30–64 with breast cancer;
California Registry, 1993

Outcome Measures	Findings

Stage of disease; mortality — Controlling for disease stage, UI had 49% higher adjusted risk of death than privately insured and Medicaid beneficiaries had a 40% higher risk of death than the privately insured 54 to 89 months after diagnosis. UI presented with later stages; Medicaid even later than uninsured

Stage of disease; mortality — Indigent patients had poorer survival rates than the privately insured for every cancer type. In the first 5 years, indigent patients did substantially worse than the privately insured in short-term survival and prognosis. Least difference was found between privately insured and indigent when chance of survival was either excellent or poor

Stage of disease — UI more likely than those with indemnity coverage to have a late-stage diagnosis (OR = 1.6 in bivariate analysis). In mulitvariate analysis OR = 1.49 (CI: 0.88–2.50). Race and SES are not independently associated with later-stage diagnoses

5-year cancer survival rate — Residents of low-income areas in Honolulu had worse cancer survival than those in Toronto; no difference in survival rates for residents of high-income areas in the two cities. Data are not sufficient to attribute differences to health insurance. Omitted variable bias potentially great

Stage of disease; selected treatment; mortality over 4–10-yr follow-up — Publicly insured and uninsured combined have OR of 2.0 for late-stage diagnosis and a relative risk of death from breast cancer of 1.42, all causes RR = 1.46. For UI, quality of life 2 years after diagnosis is worse in some domains

Health-related quality of life — Health insurance independently affects HRQOL over time in men treated for prostate cancer. Clinical and SES adjustments

Stage at diagnosis — Late-stage disease at diagnosis is more likely for those Medi-Cal enrollees who did not have benefits prior to diagnosis (OR = 3.89 compared with non-Medi-Cal women; OR = 1.39 for those with Medi-Cal in year prior to diagnosis). 18% of Medi-Cal women diagnosed with breast cancer were UI during year before diagnosis

Sample Size/Data Source

Roetzheim et al. (1999) Effects of Health Insurance and Race on Early Detection of Cancer. *J Natl Cancer Inst*	34,616 cases of colorectal, breast, and prostate cancer and melanoma; 1994 Florida Cancer Data System
Roetzheim et al. (2000b) Effects of Health Insurance and Race on Colorectal Cancer Treatments and Outcomes. *Am J Pub Health*	9,551 cases of colorectal cancer; 1994 Florida Cancer Data System
Roetzheim et al. (2000a) Effects of Health Insurance and Race on Breast Carcinoma Treatments and Outcomes. *Cancer*	11,113 cases of female breast carcinoma; 1994 Florida Cancer Data System

Chronic Diseases

General

Ayanian et al. (2000) Unmet Health Needs of Uninsured Adults in the United States. *JAMA*	105,764 adults 18–64 (1997); 117,364 (1998); BRFSS
Curtis et al. (1997) Absence of Health Insurance Is Associated with Decreased Life Expectancy in Patients with Cystic Fibrosis. *Am J Respir Crit Care Med*	189 patients with cystic fibrosis born 1955–1970 hospitalized at teaching hospital in Washington

Outcome Measures	Findings

Stage of disease

UI had greater chance than privately insured of late-stage diagnosis for colon cancer (OR = 1.67); melanoma (OR = 2.59); breast cancer (OR = 1.43) and prostate cancer (OR = 1.47). Medicaid patients had ORs (compared to privately insured) for melanoma and breast cancer of 4.69 and 1.87, respectively. SES measures gathered at population level, not individual patient level

Treatment type; mortality over 36–48 month followup

UI had higher risk of dying than private FFS patients, even adjusting for stage at diagnosis and therapy (RR = 1.41). UI patients were significantly less likely than private FFS patients to receive definitive surgery (OR = 0.57) but not less likely to be treated with chemotherapy or radiation

Mortality over 36–38-month follow-up

Relationship between health insurance and mortality (UI to FFS, RR = 1.31) is due to stage at diagnosis. Race is associated with survival after controlling for diagnosis stage and treatment modality. UI less likely than FFS to get breast-conserving surgery (OR = 0.70). Longitudinal follow-up. Same data set as in Roetzheim et al. (1999)

Multiple measures of access; self-reported health status; use of preventive services and chronic disease care

Long-term UI (≥1 year) adults reported much greater unmet health needs than insured adults. Long-term and short-term (<1 year) UI adults were more likely than insured adults to report they could not see a physician when needed due to cost (26.8%, 21.7%, and 8.2%, respectively), especially among those in poor health (69.1%, 51.9%, and 21.8%) or fair health (48.8%, 42.4%, and 15.7%). Long-term UI adults were much more likely than short-term UI and insured adults not to have had a routine check-up in the last 2 years (42.8%, 22.3%, and 17.8%). Deficits in cancer screening, cardiovascular risk reduction, and diabetes were more pronounced among long-term UI adults than among short-term UI or insured adults

Survival from birth

Median survival of insured (private and Medicaid), 20.5 years; of uninsured, 6.1 years. RR of death for uninsured to private = 2.1. HI and SES independently associated with longer survival

Sample Size/Data Source

Fish-Parcham (2001)   1996 MEPS and NHANES III; persons <65
Getting Less Care: The Uninsured With
Chronic Health Conditions. Families USA

Karlson et al. (1995)   99 SLE patients
The Independence and Stability of
Socieconomic Predictors of Morbidity
in Systemic Lupus Erythematosus (SLE).
Arthritis and Rheumatism

Asthma

Apter et al. (1999)   50 patients with moderate to severe asthma, 1991
The Influence of Demographic and
Socioeconomic Factors on Health-Related
Quality of Life in Asthma. *J Aller*
Clin Immunol

DeCorte et al. (1995)   120,032 persons with asthma; NHIS, 1991
Health Insurance: Impact on
Hospitalization Rates for Asthma.
Nursingconnections

Haas et al. (1994)   97 patients 18–55 yrs in one Boston hospital,
The Impact of Socioeconomic Status on   1989–1990
the Intensity of Ambulatory Treatment
and Health Outcomes After Hospital
Discharge for Adults with Asthma.
J Gen Intern Med

Nauenberg and Basu (1999)   1,240 asthma admissions; Los Angeles, CA,
Effect of Insurance Coverage on the   1991–1994
Relationship Between Asthma
Hospitalizations and Exposure to Air
Pollution. *Public Health Rep*

Hypertension

Ford et al. (1998)   1,724 women 50–64 yrs, NHANES III,
Health Insurance Status and   1988–1994
Cardiovascular Disease Risk Factors
Among 50–64-Year-Old U.S. Women:
Findings from the Third National
Health and Nutrition Examination
Survey. *J Women's Health*

Outcome Measures	Findings
Multiple measures of access; utilization; health status	UI with chronic conditions receive less care than those with any HI. Those with heart disease: 28% fewer visits. Hypertension: 26% fewer visits. Arthritis: 27% fewer visits. Back pain: 19% fewer visits. UI less likely to have RSC both overall and for those with specific chronic conditions. Cost is barrier for UI to getting care. UI with chronic conditions less likely to have had laboratory services appropriate for condition within the past year
Disease activity; progression of SLE; morbidity	Private HI or Medicare and greater educational attainment were independent predictors of lesser disease severity at diagnosis. Very small and nonrepresentative sample; multiple hypotheses
Health-related quality of life; asthma severity	Severity, race–ethnicity, and SES (including HI status) related to HRQOL. Individual contributing factors confounded in study. Small sample
Hospitalization	9.7% of UI with asthma were hospitalized compared to 7.1% of those with private health insurance. Lower-income people were more likely to be hospitalized than those of higher or middle income regardless of insurance status
Severity of illness; source of care; intensity of therapy; health outcome	SES and race primary focus of study. More intensive therapy was associated with improved outcomes. Lower-SES adults have greater severity of illness and less intensive therapy. UI and Medicaid patients less likely to receive intensive therapy than privately insured patients (42%, 29%, and 72%, respectively)
Hospital admissions for asthma in central Los Angeles	Only Medi-Cal admissions related to increased hospitalizations during periods of higher air pollution. UI and all other insurance not correlated with higher air pollution and higher admissions
Cardiovascular risk profile (behaviors and outcomes)	UI women had worse cardiovascular risk profile and used services less frequently. Race and education accounted for effect of HI status for physical activity, alcohol use, and hypertension

Sample Size/Data Source

Huttin et al. (2000)
Patterns and Cost for Hypertension
Treatment in the United States.
Clinical Drug Investigations

6,398 adults >18 yrs diagnosed with
hypertension; NMES, 1987

Keeler et al. (1985)
How Free Care Reduced Hypertension
in the Health Insurance Experiment.
JAMA

3,958 adults 14–61 yrs in RAND HIE,
1974–1982

Lurie et al. (1984)
Lurie et al. (1986)
(See description in General Health
Outcomes section above).

Shea et al. (1992b) Predisposing Factors
for Severe, Uncontrolled Hypertension
in an Inner-City Minority Population.
N Engl J Med

93 Black and Hispanic patients with severe
uncontrolled hypertension, 114 control
patients with hypertension, 2 New York
City hospitals 1989–1991

Shea et al. (1992a)
Correlates of Nonadherence to
Hypertension Treatment in an
Inner-City Minority Population.
Am J Pub Health

202 black and Hispanic patients; 87 who were
more adherent to drug treatment for
hypertension, 115 less adherent

Wang and Stafford (1998)
National Patterns and Predictors of
Beta-Blocker Use in Patients With
Coronary Artery Disease. *Arch Intern Med*

11,745 office visits by patients with CAD.
1993–1996

Outcome Measures	Findings

Therapy without
hypertensive medication;
no. of medications; costs
of treatment

Compared to UI those with Medicaid, Medicare +
Medicaid, private insurance, and Medicare + private
insurance were more likely to receive an Rx (ORs = 2.26,
1.95, 1.59, and 2.63, respectively). Those with Medicare
only (no supplemental coverage) are no more likely to
receive a prescription than UI (UI = UI for full year).
Detailed HI categories

Diastolic blood pressure

For clinically defined hypertensives, patients with free care
had significantly lower BP than those with cost sharing
(differential = 1.9 mm Hg). Larger difference for low-
income patients than high income (3.5 vs. 1.1 mm Hg). No
differences between blacks and whites. Authors attribute
differences in rates of diagnosis and effective treatment to
more frequent physician visits in free-care group. Also
higher patient compliance with prescription therapy and
behavioral modifications in free-care group

Hypertensive emergency

Case control study. In model adjusted for sociodemographic
factors and smoking, uninsured are more likely to have
severe uncontrolled hypertension than those with any
insurance (OR = 2.2). Not having an RSC is even more
predictive of uncontrolled hypertension (OR = 4.4). HI
status and RSC not included in same model. When single
model contained RSC, HI status, and noncompliance with
therapy, UI was no longer significant (OR = 1.9; CI:
0.8–4.6)

Nonadherence to BP
medication

Poor adherence associated with no RSC and having BP
checked in ED. UI not significantly associated with outcome
in bivariate or multivariate analyses (OR = 1.6, CI:
0.84–3.1)

Beta-blocker use

Compared to all others, privately insured more likely to
ceive beta-blocker (OR = 1.22, CI: 0.96–1.56). Uninsured
and publicly insured combined

Sample Size/Data Source

Diabetes

Beckles et al. (1998)   2,118 adults age ≥18 yrs; BRFSS, 1994
Population-Based Assessment of the
Level of Care Among Adults with
Diabetes in the U.S. *Diabetes Care*

Palta et al. (1997)   577 new diabetes cases <30 yrs of age in
Risk Factors for Hospitalization in a   Wisconsin, 1987–1992
Cohort with Type 1 Diabetes.
Am J Epidemiology

Ruggiero et al. (1997)   2,056 adults: 988 diabetics in
Diabetes Self-Management. *Diabetes Care*   representative sample; 1,068 diabetic insulin
                                               takers in augmented sample (no date)

Schiff et al. (1998)   218 adults with diabetes at one public hospital
Access to Primary Care for Patients   clinic in Chicago
with Diabetes at an Urban Public
Hospital Walk-in Clinic. *J Health
Care Poor Underserved*

End-Stage Renal Disease

Kausz et al. (2000)   90,897 adults initiating ESRD dialysis;
Late Initiation of Dialysis Among   USRDS, 1995–1997
Women and Ethnic Minorities in the
United States. *J Am Soc Nephrology*

Krop et al. (1999)   1,434 adults 45–64 with diabetes
A Community-Based Study of
Explanatory Factors for the Excess
Risk for Early Renal Function Decline
in Blacks vs. Whites with Diabetes.
Arch Intern Med

Outcome Measures	Findings

Preventive and routine care for diabetes

UI adults with diabetes are less likely to receive preventive and routine services for this condition. UI vs. insured insulin users are less likely to self-monitor blood glucose (OR = 0.3, CI: 0.1–1.25) or to receive foot exam (OR = 0.25) or eye exam (OR = 0.34). For nonusers of insulin, UI less likely to self-monitor blood glucose (OR = 0.5), receive foot exam (OR = 2.57), or have a dilated eye exam (OR = 0.5)

Hospitalization for conditions related to diabetes

Significantly higher hospital use for first 18-months postdiagnosis for Medicaid or uninsured vs. privately insured patients (RR = 2.1)

Self-monitored blood glucose; diet; exercise

No differences among HI status categories in self-management practices

Regular primary care source, diabetes care contingent on RPCS

UI patients were significantly less likely to have a RPCS than insured patients (OR = 0.37). UI received significantly fewer components of routine diabetes care within study period than insured patients (3.4 vs. 4.3 components). Patients with RPCS received significantly more components of care than those without RPCS (4.2 vs. 3.2)

Late initiation of dialysis as measured by clinical factor (glomerular filtration rate <5ml/min)

Compared to those with any kind of insurance prior to initiation of dialysis, UI were more likely to begin dialysis at a clinically late stage (OR = 1.55)

Early renal function decline as measured by increased serum creatinine

Over 3-year follow-up blacks were more likely to develop early renal function decline than whites (OR = 3.15). Overall, in bivariate analysis, UI had a greater risk of early renal function decline (OR = 2.0). Controlling for education, income, health insurance, glucose level, BP, smoking, and physical activity reduced the excess risk for blacks by 82% (OR = 1.38, CI: 0.71–2.69)

Sample Size/Data Source

Obrador et al. (1999)
Prevalence of and Factors Associated
with Suboptimal Care Before Initiation
of Dialysis in the United States.
J Ame Soc Nephrology

155,076 adults starting ESRD dialysis,
USRDS, 1995–1997

Powe et al. (1999)
Septicemia in Dialysis Patients: Incidence,
Risk Factors, and Prognosis. *Kidney
Int*

USRDS hospitalization and death records
over 7 yrs

HIV

Andersen et al. (2000)
Access of Vulnerable Groups to
Antiretroviral Therapy Among Persons
in Care for HIV Disease in the United
States. *Health Serv Res*

2,776 HIV+ adults under treatment; HCSUS

Bennett et al. (1995)
Racial Differences in Care Among
Hospitalized Patients with
Pneumocystis carinii Pneumonia in
Chicago, New York, Los Angeles,
Miami, and Raleigh-Durham.
Arch Intern Med

1,547 HIV+ patients in non-VA hospitals in
5 cities, 1987–1990

Bing et al. (1999)
Protease Inhibitor Use Among a
Community Sample of People with
HIV Disease. *J Acquire Immune
Defic Syndr*

1,034 HIV+ adult clients of an HIV/AIDS
community services organization

Cunningham et al. (1995)
Access to Medical Care and Health-
Related Quality of Life for Low-Income
Persons With Symptomatic Human
Immunodeficiency Virus. *Med Care*

205 patients in one VA hospital and one
public hospital

Outcome Measures	Findings

Pre-ESRD care; morbidity; mortality; resource utilization

Population of those entering Medicare (ESRD) system. Uninsured patients sicker, less likely to have received EPO prior to dialysis. UI had worst outcomes, followed by Medicaid beneficiaries. Compared with privately insured, UI were less likely to have received EPO (OR = 0.49); Medicaid to privately insured for EPO: OR = 0.66. Compared to those with private insurance prior to ESRD, UI were more likely to have hypoalbuminemia (OR = 1.37) and a hematocrit <28% (OR = 1.34)

Hospital admission for septicemia; mortality

Relative risk of septicemia in peritoneal dialysis patients is 2.69 for UI compared with Medicare and privately insured patients. RR = 1.83 for Medicaid vs. Medicare and private. No statistically significant differences among hemodialysis patients. ESRD patients with septicemia had twice the risk of death of those without this complication. Differing results by type of dialysis are hard to interpret. Authors suggest patients present with more advanced disease and have already suffered adverse effects of uremia, hypertension, and hyperparathyroidism

Receipt of HAART by end of 1996

Fully adjusted, uninsured were less likely to receive HAART than privately insured, but this was not statistically significant (OR = 0.74, CI not given). Need for HAART defined by low CD4 count

In-hospital mortality; bronchoscopy

Uninsured had higher in-hospital mortality rate than privately insured in non-VA facilities (OR = 1.5). Medicaid also had a higher mortality rate than privately insured (OR = 2.1) in non-VA hospitals. UI as likely as privately insured to receive bronchoscopy in non-VA hospitals

Use of protease inhibitors

UI are less likely to use PIs than privately insured patients and those who pay out of pocket (OR = 1.57, CI: 0.96–2.5). Poor response rate

HRQOL; access to care

Patients with higher access scores report significantly better HRQOL scores, freedom from pain, emotional well-being, and hopefulness. UI reported significantly worse overall perceived access than Medi-Cal patients. Also reported more problems meeting costs of care than either Medi-Cal or VA patients. Compared with Medi-Cal, UI went without care more often because of cost. Compared with VA patients, UI had more problems being admitted to the hospital and getting emergency care

Sample Size/Data Source

Cunningham et al. (1996)
Access to Community-Based Medical
Services and Number of Hospitalizations
Among Patients with HIV Disease:
Are They Related? *J Acquired Immune
Defic Syndr Hum Retrovirol*

217 patients in 7 California hospitals

Cunningham et al. (1999)
The Impact of Competing Subsistence
Needs and Barriers on Access to Medical
Care for Persons With Human
Immunodefiency Virus Receiving Care
in the United States. *Med Care*

2,864 adults receiving HIV care, HCSUS
1996–1997

Cunningham et al. (2000)
Prevalence and Predictors of Highly
Active Antiretroviral Therapy Use in
Patients with HIV Infection in the
United States. *J Acquire Immune
Defic Syndr*

(Same sample as above)

Fleishman and Mor (1993)
Insurance Status Among People With
AIDS: Relationships With
Sociodemographic Characteristics and
Service Use. *Inquiry*

937 AIDS patients in 9 communities;
ACSUS, 1988–1989

Goldman et al. (2001)
Effect of Insurance on Mortality in an
HIV-Positive Population in Care.
J American Statistical Assoc

2,864 HIV+ patients; HCSUS, 1996–1998

Joyce et al. (1999)
Variation in Inpatient Resource Use in
the Treatment of HIV. *Med Care*

1,949 HIV+ patients in 10 cities, 1991–1992

Katz et al. (1992)
CD4 Lymphocyte Count as an Indicator
of Delay in Seeking Human
Immunodeficiency Virus-Related
Treatment. *Arch Intern Med*

96 patients in a university clinic, 1989–1991

Outcome Measures	Findings

Access to care	Those hospitalized with HIV were asked to rate their ability to get outpatient care in the community prior to their first hospitalization for HIV, with 0 = lack of access and 100 = highest possible access. UI had a mean score of 57, Medi-Cal beneficiaries, 59, VA 60, and private insurance, 69. Only one very global question was used to assess access
Receipt of needed care	Same sample as Andersen et al. (2000), Cunningham et al. (2000). In unadjusted, bivariate analyses, 19.1% of UI vs. 9.6% of insured went without care for HIV because they needed money for basic necessities. 45% of UI vs. 34% of insured postponed care because of one or more competing needs. Both findings statistically significant
Receipt of HAART	Follow-up of Andersen et al. (2000) one year later. UI significantly less likely to receive HAART at follow-up than privately insured FFS patients (OR = 0.71)
Site of care; hospital admission; LOS; ED visits	95% of the UI and the publicly insured vs. 47% of the privately insured used hospital clinics as their source of medical care for AIDS. UI were less likely than those with private insurance to have been admitted overnight to a hospital, their LOS was shorter, and they had fewer outpatient visits. No difference in ED visits depending on insurance status. Convenience sample
Mortality	HI is associated with a lower 6-month mortality rate. For those interviewed in 1996, mortality was 71% lower for those with HI compared to UI. For those interviewed in 1997 when drug therapies were more widely used, insured patients had an 85% lower mortality rate than UI
Hospital admission; LOS; hospital charge	Medicaid enrollees with HIV are more likely to be admitted to private hospitals than UI and those covered by other public programs. Privately insured patients are most likely to be admitted to private hospitals. 63% of UI patients admitted to public hospitals, compared with 39% of Medicaid patients and 16% of privately insured patients. Per diem charges significantly lower for UI than for private insured and total charges even within hospital are significantly lower for UI
CD4 lymphocyte count	Patients with private insurance had significantly lower CD4 lymphocyte counts (worse outcome) than patients with public insurance. UI patients had intermediate counts between the privately and publicly insured. Hypothesis is that patients with private coverage were reluctant to use it and may have misrepresented HI status.

Sample Size/Data Source

Katz et al. (1995)
Health Insurance and Use of Medical
Services by Men Infected With HIV.
*J Acquir Immune Defic Syndr Hum
Retrovir*

178 HIV+ men recruited from one clinic, 1991

Mor et al. (1992)
Variations in Health Services Use
Among HIV-Infected Patients. *Med Care*

Same as Fleishman and Mor (1993)

Niemcryk et al. (1998)
Consistency in Maintaining Contact
with HIV-Related Service Providers:
An Analysis of the AIDS Cost and
Services Utilization Study (ACSUS).
J Community Health

Same as Joyce et al. (1999)

Palacio et al. (1999)
Access to and Utilization of Primary
Care Services Among HIV-Infected
Women. *J Acquir Immune Defic Syndr*

213 HIV+ women in telephone survey

Shapiro et al. (1999)
Variations in the Care of HIV-Infected
Adults in the United States. *JAMA*

2,864 HIV+ respondents in HCSUS, 1996–1998

Sorvillo et al. (1999)
Use of Protease Inhibitors Among
Persons with AIDS in Los Angeles
County. *AIDS Care*

339 HIV+ men and women in Los Angeles
County, 1996–1997

Outcome Measures	Findings

Outpatient visits; PCP prophylaxis use

UI men had significantly fewer outpatient visits and fewer ED visits than men with FFS or managed care insurance. Use of PCP prophylaxis was similar for those with FFS (93%) and managed care (83%) but lower for UI (63%). Having private insurance resulted in higher use of outpatient services

Hospital admissions; outpatient and clinic visits; ED visits; site of care

UI were less likely than those with public insurance to use the ED (30% vs. 46%) and more likely than the privately insured (24%). UI were less likely to have been hospitalized than those either with public insurance or private insurance (18%, 39%, and 27%, respectively). UI had fewer outpatient visits annually than either publicly or privately insured

ED visits; hospital admission; use of ambulatory care

Having had a visit at a previous time increases the probability of later visits. People with Medicaid and other public assistance (UI) more likely to be hospitalized than people with private insurance

Primary care provider; No. of primary care visits; missed appointments

Lack of any insurance is significantly associated with missing one or more primary care service appointments (OR = 2.76), but not with having a primary care provider or number of visits. Small number of uninsured (n = 37)

6 measures of access to care; service use and medications

Care received by both UI and Medicaid patients was less than that received by privately insured on 5 of 6 access measures. Wait for starting PI and NRRTI treatment ranged from 9.4 months for privately insured to 12.4 months for Medicaid beneficiaries to 13.9 months for UI. Unadjusted, 21% of UI patients had <2 visits within 6 months, compared with 16% of Medicaid and 12–13% of patients with private insurance or Medicare. UI more likely than privately insured to have ED visit without hospitalization in 6 months (OR = 1.45); and less likely to have ever received antiretroviral treatment (OR = 0.35)

Use of protease inhibitors

Use of PIs more common for the insured (67%) than the uninsured (49%). Controlling for site of care (private clinic, HMO, public clinic) eliminated significance of HI status

Sample Size/Data Source

Turner et al. (2000)
Delayed Medical Care After Diagnosis
in a US National Probability Sample
of Persons Infected with Human
Immunodeficiency Virus. *Arch Intern Med*

2 overlapping cohorts of 1,540 and 1,960
HIV+ patients; HCSUS, 1993–1996

Mental Illness

Cooper-Patrick et al. (1999)
Mental Health Service Utilization by
African-Americans and Whites: The
Baltimore Epidemiological Catchment
Area Followup. *Med Care*

1,662 adults in longitudinal study in Baltimore,
Maryland, 1981–1996

Druss and Rosenheck (1998)
Mental Disorders and Access to Medical
Care in the United States. *Am J Psych*

77,183 adult respondents to the 1994 NHIS;
7,409 reporting mental disorder

McAlpine and Mechanic (2000)
Utilization of Specialty Mental Health
Care Among Persons with Severe
Mental Illness: The Roles of
Demographics, Need, Insurance, and
Risk. *Health Serv Res*

9,585 adults 18–97 yrs from 60 communities,
1997–1998

Rabinowitz et al. (1998)
Relationship Between Type of Insurance
and Care During Early Course of
Psychosis. *Am J Psych*

514 patients with psychosis in 12 psychiatric
facilities in Suffolk County, New York,
1989–1995

(Same Database)

Rabinowitz et al. (2001)
Changes in Insurance Coverage and
Extent of Care During the Two Years
After First Hospitalization for a Psychotic
Disorder. *Psych Services*

443 patients 15–60 yrs in 12 psychiatric
facilities in Suffolk County, New York,
1989–1995

Outcome Measures   Findings

3-6 month delay in treatment   In bivariate analysis, 22–37% of UI delayed treatment >3
after diagnosis   months after diagnosis, compared with 14–25% of privately
                                   insured and 9–19% of Medicaid patients. Delays in care
                                   diminished for newly diagnosed at later time (1995). In
                                   multivariable analysis, RSC was significant predictor of less
                                   delay in care; UI no longer significant as predictor of delay
                                   compared with privately insured (OR = 1.28, CI: 0.84–1.93)

Use of mental health services   Mental health service use increased over course of the study
in 6 months prior to   by both blacks and whites. Increase in use by blacks achieved
interview   predominantly in the general medical sector. Overall, and
                                   separately for blacks, being UI decreased the likelihood of
                                   receiving mental health services compared with having health
                                   insurance in a multivariable analysis (ORs = 0.63 for
                                   everyone and 0.45 for blacks)

Receipt of care for reported   Persons with mental illness are as likely as those without this
mental disorder   disorder to have health insurance and an RSC, but were more
                                   likely to have been denied insurance because of preexisting
                                   condition. Persons with a mental disorder were more likely
                                   to have delayed care because of cost (OR = 1.76) and were
                                   less likely to be able to obtain needed care (OR = 0.43)

Severe mental illness;   In bivariate analysis, severely mentally ill and less severely ill
outpatient specialty mental   were more likely to be uninsured than those without any
health care   measured mental disorder. Among persons with severe mental
                                   illness, UI were much less likely to have used specialty mental
                                   health care than people with public insurance (OR = 0.17)
                                   and less likely than those with private insurance to use
                                   specialty care as well (OR = 0.4)

Preadmission treatment;   Over 24 months, the publicly insured had the most days of
clinical treatment; outpatient   care, the privately insured the least inpatient care. Those with
treatment   no insurance were less likely to receive outpatient care than
                                   either the privately or the publicly insured (ORs = 0.53 and
                                   0.56, respectively)

Inpatient, outpatient, and day   Many people change health insurance status over time after
hospital care; change in   first hospital visit for mental illness. 54% of UI at baseline
health insurance status   obtained coverage by 24 months. Over 24 months, Medicaid
                                   and Medicare patients had more days of care, privately insured
                                   had least inpatient care, and uninsured were least likely to
                                   receive outpatient care. Study suggests systematic changes in
                                   health insurance over the course of mental illness

Sample Size/Data Source

Sturm and Wells (2000)   9,585 respondents to HealthCare for
Health Insurance May Be Improving—   Communities national survey, 1996, 1998
But Not for Individuals With Mental
Illness. *Health Serv Res*

Wang et al. (2000)   3,032 respondents, Midlife Development in
Recent Care of Common Mental   the United States survey, 1996
Disorders in the United States. *J Gen*
Intern Med

Young et al. (2001)   1,636 adults with provable depressive
The Quality of Care for Depressive   disorder in telephone survey, 1997
and Anxiety Disorders in the United
States. *Arch Gen Psych*

Hospital Care

Broyles et al. (2000)   1,512 adults in Oklahoma, 1993 BRFSS
Equity Concerns with the Use of
Hospital Services by the Medically
Vulnerable. *J Health Care Poor Underserved*

Burstin et al. (1992)   31,249 patient records from acute care hospitals
Socioeconomic Status and Risk for   in New York, 1984
Substandard Medical Care. *JAMA*

Greenberg et al. (1988)   1,403 patients 31-93 yrs in New Hampshire
Social and Economic Factors in the   and Vermont, 1973–1976
Choice of Lung Cancer Treatment.
N Engl J Med

Hadley et al. (1991)   592,598 patients <65 hospitalized in 1987 in a
Comparison of Uninsured and   national sample of hospitals
Privately Insured Hospital Patients. *JAMA*

Kerr and Siu (1993)   50 patients meeting criteria admitted through
Follow-up After Hospital Discharge: ED to teaching hospital, 1990
Does Insurance Make a Difference?
J Health Care Poor Underserved

Outcome Measures	Findings

Mental health status; probable depressive disorder; access to care

Adults with a probable mental health disorder are more likely to have lost HI in the previous year than those without a disorder and are more likely to report difficulty in getting care

Receipt of any mental health care and guideline-concordant care

Specifically asked about HI coverage for mental health care, not general HI. Having insurance for mental health services predicted overall likelihood of therapy, therapy in mental health sector, and guideline-concordant treatment (ORs = 2.3, 3.2, and 2.8–4.2, respectively)

Self-reported use of health services; receipt of appropriate care

Contact with provider (any kind) less likely for UI (OR = 0.46), but type of or presence of insurance had no effect on receipt of appropriate care for anxiety or depression

Hospital admission; LOS

Uninsured patients in fair or poor health were significantly less likely than uninsured in better health to be hospitalized and had significantly shorter LOS

Adverse events due to negligence

Uninsured had greater risk of substandard care than privately insured (OR = 2.35). Medicaid patients had insignificantly different risk from privately insured. UI patients most likely to experience injury due to substandard care in emergency department. ED is disproportionately the site of care for UI patients. Hospital-level variables controlled for

Treatment type; mortality

Medicare–Medicaid–UI grouped together and were less likely to have surgery than privately insured; no difference in mortality

In-hospital mortality; use of specific procedures; biopsy results

In 10 of 16 age, sex, and race-specific cohorts (8 of 12 for adults), UI had a higher risk of in-hospital death than did privately insured after adjusting for severity at admission (RRs range from 1.1 to 3.2). UI were less likely to undergo high-cost or discretionary procedures and less likely to have normal biopsy results for 5 of 7 endoscopic procedures

Follow-up care

Medicaid and UI patients were significantly less likely to receive follow-up care than Medicare and privately insured patients. UI and Medicaid patients were also less likely to have a regular physician or complete specific discharge instructions. Cost of care was found to be the most significant deterrent to receiving follow-up care

Sample Size/Data Source

Schnitzler et al. (1998)
Variations in Healthcare Measures by
Insurance Status for Patients Receiving
Ventilator Support. *Clin Perform
Qual Health Care*

21,149 hospital patients; HCUP data, 1989-1992

Weissman and Epstein (1989)
Case Mix and Resource Utilization by
Uninsured Hospital Patients in the
Boston Metropolitan Area. *JAMA*

65,032 patients <65 from 52 hospitals in
Boston, 1983

Weissman et al. (1991)
Delayed Access to Health Care: Risk
Factors, Reasons, and Consequences.
Ann Intern Med

12,068 adult patients hospitalized in 5
Massachusetts hospitals 1987

Weissman et al. (1994)
The Impact of Patient Socioeconomic
Status and Other Social Factors on
Readmission: A Prospective Study in
Four Massachusetts Hospitals. *Inquiry*

10,158 adult patients hospitalized in 4
Massachusetts hospitals, 1987

Yelin et al. (1983)
Is Health Care Use Equivalent Across
Social Groups? A Diagnosis-Based Study.
Am J Public Health

1,788 participants, 1976 NHIS

Yergan et al. (1988)
Relationship Between Patient Source of
Payment and the Intensity of
Hospital Services. *Med Care*

4,369 inpatients with pneumonia in 17
randomly selected hospitals, 1970–1973

Outcome Measures	Findings

In-hospital mortality; no. of procedures; LOS; charges

Mortality rates for privately insured (FFS) were 30% and for Medicaid patients were 28%; for UI 27%; for Medicare 26%; and for HMO or PHP, 26%. For-profit hospitals had significantly higher mortality rates than not-for-profit hospitals. UI had 16% shorter LOS and Medicaid patients 10% longer LOS than FFS in a multivariable analysis. HMO, UI, Medicaid, and Medicare patients all had more procedures than FFS patients

Severity of illness; no. of procedures; LOS

UI had 7% shorter stays and underwent 7% fewer procedures than Blue Cross patients, with differences varying by hospital type. Compared to Medicaid patients, they had shorter stays on average (5.4 vs. 5.9 days), but underwent a similar number of procedures. Adjusted for case mix, severity of UI patients was 30% higher in public hospitals and 8% higher in teaching hospitals compared with other institutions. Across all hospitals, UI and Blue Cross patients had similar severity

Delays in care; LOS

Delays in care led to longer LOS. 24% of UI patients delayed obtaining care (OR = 1.7) compared to 23% of Medicaid (OR = 1.6), 15% of Medicare (OR = 0.9), 18% of HMO (OR=1.2), and 16% of Blue Cross or commercial, the comparison group

Readmission to hospital at 7 and 60 days after discharge

UI were less likely than Medicaid beneficiaries or those with other insurance to be readmitted. Compared to people with private insurance, UI were less likely to be readmitted 7 days after discharge (OR = 0.36), and less likely to be readmitted 60 days after discharge (OR = 0.48). Medicaid patients were slightly more likely to be readmitted within 7 days and more likely to be readmitted in 60 days compared to privately insured (OR = 1.46)

Physician visits; condition-specific hospitalization

UI associated with lower hospitalization rates for 5 of 9 chronic conditions, symptoms, and diagnoses held constant. Overall, no consistent differences in M.D. visit rates, controlling for symptoms and diagnosis. For ill persons, UI had more M.D. visits

In-hospital mortality; ICU use; LOS

UI with pneumonia had higher mortality, higher use of ICUs, and shorter LOS. Observed-to-expected in-hospital deaths for UI = 1.38. No significant findings on service intensity. No controls for level of service

Sample Size/Data Source

Emergency and Trauma

Braveman et al. (1994) Insurance-Related Differences in the Risk of Ruptured Appendix. *N Engl J Med*	91,339 adults discharged from hospital with Dx of acute appendicitis; California, 1984–1989
Doyle (2001) Does Health Insurance Affect Treatment Decisions and Patient Outcomes? Using Automobile Accidents as Unexpected Health Shocks	10,962 accident victims <65; 1992–1997 Wisconsin's Crash Outcome Data Evaluation System
Ell et al. (1994) Acute Chest Pain in African Americans: Factors in the Delay in Seeking Emergency Care *Am J Pub Health*	254 patients at a public hospital; 194 patients at a private hospital; 1988–1990 Los Angeles
Haas and Goldman (1994) Acutely Injured Patients with Trauma in Massachusetts: Differences in Care and Mortality by Insurance Status. *Am J Pub Health*	15,008 adult trauma patients <65; Massachusetts, 1990
MacKenzie et al. (2000) Characterization of Patients With High-Energy Lower Extremity Trauma. *J Orthop Trauma*	601 patients 16–69, 8 Level I trauma centers 1994–1997
Nathens et al. (2001) Payer Status: The Unspoken Triage Criterion. *J Trauma*	2008 adults <65 King County, Washington, central region trauma registry, 1995–1998
Rhee et al. (1997) The Effect of Payer Status on Utilization of Hospital Resources in Trauma Care. *Arch Surgery*	2,827 patient data from institutional trauma registry; Washington, 1990–1992
Rucker et al. (2001) Delay in Seeking Emergency Care. *Acad Emerg Med*	1,920 patients surveyed in 5 teaching hospital EDs

Outcome Measures	Findings
Ruptured appendix	UI more likely to have a ruptured appendix compared to privately insured (OR = 1.5). Same higher risk for Medicaid compared to privately insured. UI associated with delay in seeking care
Mortality; hospital charges; LOS	UI in severe auto accidents received 20% less treatment (lower charges, shorter LOS) and had a mortality rate of 5.2% compared with 3.8% for persons with private insurance (37% higher mortality). Limited adjustment for severity
Access to care; acute chest pain; delay in seeking care	Health insurance of any kind was significantly related to decision time to seek care, but not to travel time. Those who did not go to hospital are not in study. UI associated with use of a public hospital
In-hospital mortality; receipt of services	UI receive less care and have a higher mortality rate than trauma patients with private insurance or Medicaid. They are as likely to receive care in an ICU as patients with private health insurance, but less likely to undergo an operative procedure (OR = 0.68) or receive physical therapy (OR = 0.61) and are more likely to die in the hospital (OR= 2.15)
Lower-extremity injury; amputation	Uninsured no more likely to undergo amputation. Those with this injury more likely to be uninsured than general population
Patient transfer	Medicaid and UI analyzed together. Severe injuries and "noncommercial insurance" (Medicaid and UI) most likely to be transferred to Level 1 trauma center. Controlling for age, sex, and primary injury and severity, people without commercial insurance are more likely to be transferred (OR = 2.4). Effect most pronounced for least injured
Mortality rate; LOS	Medicaid and UI combined. Payer status did not affect mortality or use of hospital resources except for one subgroup: those who required transfer to LTC. For these patients, Medicaid and UI patients had greater LOS
Self-reported delays in seeking ED care	32% of participants reported a delay in seeking ED care. Patients with no regular M.D. were more likely to delay care (OR = 2.0). UI tended to be more likely to delay care than those with any insurance, but finding was not statistically significant (OR = 1.26, CI: 0.88–1.81)

Sample Size/Data Source

Svenson and Spurlock (2001)
Insurance Status and Admission to
Hospital for Head Injuries: Are We
Part of a Two-Tiered Medical System.
Am J Emerg Med

8,591 ED patients with head injury in Kentucky

Cardiovascular Disease

Blustein et al. (1995)
Sequential Events Contributing to
Variations in Cardiac Revascularization
Rates. *Med Care*

5,857 AMI hospital admissions <65:
1991, California

Brooks et al. (2000)
The Marginal Benefits of Invasive
Treatments for Acute Myocardial
Infarction: Does Insurance Coverage
Matter? *Inquiry*

30,606 patients, HCUP data Washington,
1988–1993

Canto et al. (1999)
The Association Between the On-site
Availability of Cardiac Procedures and
the Utilization of Those Services for
Acute Myocardial Infarction by Payer
Group. *Clin Cardiol*

275,046 patients National Registry of
MI-II, 1994–1996

Canto et al. (2000)
Payer Status and the Utilization of
Hospital Resources in Acute Myocardial
Infarction. *Arch Intern Med*

332,221 patients National Registry of
Myocardial Infarction-II, 1994–1996

Carlisle et al. (1997)
Racial and Ethnic Disparities in the
Use of Cardiovascular Procedures:
Associations with Type of Health
Insurance. *Am J Pub Health*

104,952 hospital discharges in Los Angeles
county, California, 1986–1988

Carlisle and Leake (1998)
Differences in the Effect of Patients'
Socioeconomic Status on the Use of
Invasive Cardiovascular Procedures
Across Health Insurance Categories.
Am J Pub Health

206,233 discharged patients with heart
disease; California, 1991–1993

Outcome Measures	Findings

Admission to hospital; cost; LOS	Medicaid and UI less likely than privately insured with head injury to be admitted. Cost: public < uninsured < private. LOS: similar across groups. For those with less severe head injuries, insurance status is significantly associated with discretionary medical decision making in ED care. Method to adjust for severity of injury questionable
In-hospital mortality; revascularization; hospital admission	UI less likely than privately insured patients to receive revascularization at hospitals offering it (OR = 0.43 to FFS, 0.53 to HMO). Less likely to receive revascularization at every step of the care process. In-hospital death rate is higher for UI: OR = 1.13 (compared to Medicaid), 1.77 (compared to FFS), 2.07 (compared to HMO). Compared to privately insured, UI less likely to be admitted to hospital offering revascularization (OR = 0.71), less likely to be transferred to receive revascularization (OR = 0.42), and less likely to be readmitted for revascularization (OR = 0.63). Clinical adjustments; no assessment of appropriateness of procedures
Adjusted mortality at days 1, 7, 30, and 90 and at one year	Cardiac catheterization within 90 days for marginal patients in each insurance category had greater survival benefits up to 90 days for UI than for FFS, HMO, or Medicaid patients. Suggests that UI who receive the procedure are at a higher level of severity than insured patients
Coronary arteriography	UI equally likely to receive acute reperfusion therapy and less likely to undergo catheterization (OR = 0.68), PTCA (OR = 0.8), or CABG (OR = 0.78) than privately insured. Admission to hospital that offers arteriography increases likelihood of receiving it (OR for UI =1.7). Extensive adjustments for clinical factors and prior history
In-hospital mortality	In-hospital mortality for uninsured vs. FFS (OR = 1.29) is the same as Medicaid to FFS. No significant differences among in-hospital mortality rates for HMO, FFS, and Medicare
AMI, CAD, and angina	Uninsured African-American patients significantly less likely to have arteriography, CABG, or angioplasty than white UI patients (OR = 0.33–0.5). No disparities related to ethnicity in privately insured group
Angiography; CABG; angioplasty	Examined differences within insurance classes by neighborhood SES. Residents of high-SES areas were more likely and those of low-SES areas less likely to undergo each of 3 invasive procedures (angiography, CABG, angioplasty) than those of middle-SES areas. SES effects were found for Medicare and HMO patients, but were less pronounced (not significantly different) in FFS and UI patients

Sample Size/Data Source

Daumit et al. (1999)
Use of Cardiovascular Procedures
Among Black Persons and White Persons:
A 7-Year Nationwide Study in Patients
with Renal Disease. *Ann Intern Med*

4,987 adults with ESRD 1986–1987
USRDS data

Daumit et al. (2000)
Relation of Gender and Health
Insurance to Cardiovascular Procedure
Use in Persons with Progression of
Chronic Renal Disease. *Med Care*

(Same data sample as above)

Kreindel et al. (1997)
Health Insurance Coverage and
Outcome Following Acute Myocardial
Infarction: A Community-wide
Perspective. *Arch Intern Med*

3,735 AMI patients in Worcester,
Massachusetts, 1986–1993

Kuykendall et al. (1995)
Expected Source of Payment and Use
of Hospital Services for Coronary
Atherosclerosis. *Med Care*

24,424 hospital discharge abstracts,
California, 1989

Leape et al. (1999)
Underuse of Cardiac Procedures:
Do Women, Ethnic Minorities and the
Uninsured Fail to Receive Needed
Revascularization? *Ann Intern Med*

631 patients in 13 New York City
hospitals, 1992

Mancini et al. (2001)
Coronary Artery Bypass Surgery: Are
Outcomes Influenced by Demographics
or Ability to Pay? *Ann Surg*

1,556 CABG patients in single public
hospital in Los Angeles, 1990–2000

Outcome Measures	Findings

Cardiac catheterization; angioplasty; CABG — Differences between blacks and whites in use of cardiovascular procedures narrowed markedly once ESRD developed and insurance (Medicare) was universal. At baseline, UI blacks with evidence of coronary disease were much less likely to receive cardiovascular procedures than UI whites (OR = 0.07); at follow-up, previously UI black patients were slightly *more* likely to undergo a cardiac procedure than UI white patients. UI blacks and whites had the greatest disparity in the use of procedures at baseline and the largest change at follow-up, post-Medicare

Cardiac catheterization; angioplasty; CABG — Compared to men with private insurance, both women and men without insurance were less likely to receive cardiovascular procedures prior to ESRD (ORs = 0.19 and 0.47, respectively). At follow-up when everyone had Medicare (ESRD), gender differences in procedure use were eliminated for UI

In-hospital, post-AMI mortality — No significant difference in in-hospital mortality for UI to privately insured (OR = 1.21; CI: 0.60–2.44). No SES or provider adjustment

LOS; revascularization — UI patients were much less likely than FFS or HMO patients to undergo revascularization (either CABG or PTCA) (ORs = 0.46 and 0.59, respectively). UI more likely to have a longer LOS without revascularization than HMO or FFS patients (OR = 1.95). Weak adjustment for clinical factors, no adjustment for SES or provider factors. No assessment of appropriateness

CABG, PTCA — Sample consisted of patients meeting panel criteria for necessary revascularization. No difference in rates of revascularization according to HI status found in hospitals that provide CABG and coronary angioplasty. Underuse was significantly greater in hospitals without these services, particularly for UI. In these hospitals, 52% of UI received indicated procedure vs. 82% of privately insured. No significant difference in adjusted in-hospital mortality between UI and privately insured

Survival over study period — UI patients had significantly better survival at 10 years than insured patients (87% vs. 76%). No adjustment for marked differences in insured and uninsured groups, including younger age distribution of UI patients. 66% of sample was UI

Sample Size/Data Source

Sada et al. (1998)
Influence of Payor on Use of Invasive
Cardiac Procedures and Patient Outcome
After Myocardial Infarction in the
United States. *J Am Coll Cardiol*

17,600 AMI patients <65 in National
Registry of Myocardial Infarction, 1994–1995

Young and Cohen (1991)
Inequities in Hospital Care, the
Massachusetts Experience. *Inquiry*

4,972 patients admitted with AMI, 1987

Palliative Care

Holcombe and Griffin (1993)
Effect of Insurance Status on Pain
Medication Prescriptions in a
Hematology/Oncology Practice.
S Med J

710 patient charts, Louisiana State
University Medical Center, 1990

Kollef (1996)
Private Attending Physician Status and
the Withdrawal of Life-Sustaining
Interventions in a Medical Intensive
Care Unit Population. *Crit Care
Med*

Patients in the medical ICU of one
hospital, 1993–1994

Kollef and Ward (1999)
The Influence of Access to a Private
Attending Physician on the Withdrawal
of Life-Sustaining Therapies in the
Intensive Care Unit. *Critical Care Medicine*

Patients within the medical ICU of one
hospital, 1996

Ambulatory Care Sensitive Conditions

Bindman et al. (1995)
Preventable Hospitalizations and
Access to Care. *JAMA*

Telephone surveys of 6,674 adults 18–64;
mail survey of physicians in 41 areas;
1990 U.S. Census

Outcome Measures	Findings
In-hospital mortality; nondiscretionary angiography; LOS	UI less likely than FFS patients to receive nondiscretionary angiography (OR = 0.48). Payer status not associated with length of stay. Medicaid patients had higher mortality than FFS
Mortality in hospital and at 30 days post-discharge. Receipt of invasive cardiac procedures	UI had higher 30-day postdischarge mortality relative to FFS (OR = 1.6) and HMO (OR = 1.5). Compared with FFS, UI were less likely to receive 2 of 3 cardiac procedures (CABG and angioplasty) (OR = 0.6). Compared to HMO patients, UI were about equally likely to receive arteriography and CABG, but less likely to receive angioplasty (OR = 0.6). No assessment of procedure appropriateness; no validation of AMI diagnosis or clinical covariates
Receipt of pain medication; class of pain medication	Medicaid outpatients are more likely to receive any pain medications than UI or Medicare patients. Also more likely to receive longer-lasting, more efficacious, and more expensive pain medications
Withdrawal of life support; duration of mechanical ventilation; ICU LOS; medical care costs; patient charges	Having private HI and private attending M.D. are correlated. Patients without private HI (Medicaid and UI) are more likely to have life-sustaining treatment withdrawn (OR = 4.4) than are privately insured
Access to a private attending M.D.	Having a private M.D. is strongly associated with no withdrawal of care. Private insurance is strongly associated with having a private M.D. (OR = 3.5)
Preventable hospitalizations	Access to care and area-wide rates of uninsured were inversely related to hospitalization rate for five chronic conditions: asthma, hypertension, CHF, COPD, and diabetes. Authors hypothesize that even acutely ill UI are less likely to seek care. Ecological findings

Sample Size/Data Source

Gaskin and Hoffman (2000) Racial and Ethnic Differences in Preventable Hospitalizations Across 10 States. *Med Care Res Rev*	1996 hospital discharge data from 10 states representing 42% of U.S. population
Weissman et al. (1992) Rates of Avoidable Hospitalization by Insurance Status in Massachusetts and Maryland. *JAMA*	Massachusetts and Maryland hospital discharges for patients <65, 1987

NOTES: ACSUS = AIDS Cost and Services Utilization Study; AMI = acute myocardial infarction; AOR = adjusted odds ratio; BP = blood pressure; BRFSS = Behavioral Risk Factor Surveillance System; CABG = coronary artery bypass graft; CAD = coronary artery disease; CBE = clinical breast exam; CHF = congestive heart failure; CI = confidence interval; COPD = chronic obstructive pulmonary disease; DRE = digital rectal examination; Dx = diagnosis; ED = emergency department; EPO = erythropoietin; ESRD = end-stage renal disease; FFS = fee for service; FOBT = fecal occult blood test; FPL = federal poverty level; HAART = highly active antiretroviral therapy; HCSUS = HIV Cost and Services Utilization Study; HCUP = Healthcare Cost and Utilization Project; HI = health insurance; HIE = Health Insurance Experiment (RAND); HMO = health maintenance organization; HRQOL = health–related quality of life; ICU = intensive care unit; LOS = length of stay; LTC = long-term care; MH = mental health; MIDUS = Midlife Development in the

Outcome Measures	Findings
Preventable hospitalizations	Analysis was stratified by health insurance status, thus no direct comparison by HI status made. Within classes of HI status, blacks and Hispanics more likely to have preventable hospitalizations
Preventable hospitalizations	In Massachusetts, hospitalization rates for uninsured and privately insured were significantly different for 10 of 12 conditions. In Maryland, for 9 of 12 conditions. UI and Medicaid patients more likely than privately insured to be hospitalized (ORs = 1.3–1.7 for UI compared to private, and 1.3–1.7 for Medicaid compared to private)

United States; NHANES = National Health and Nutrition Examination Survey; NHIS = National Health Interview Survey; NMES = National Medical Expenditures Survey; NNRTI = nonnucleoside reverse transcriptase inhibitor; NSD = no significant difference; OR = odds ratio; PCP = *Pneumocystis carinii* pneumonia; PHP = prepaid health plan ; PI = protease inhibitor; PSA = prostate-specific antigen; PTCA = percutaneous transluminal coronary angioplasty; QOL = quality of life; RPCS = regular primary care source; RR = relative risk; RSC = regular source of care; Rx = prescription medication; SES = socioeconomic status; SLE = systemic lupus erythematosus; SMR = standardized mortality ratio; Tx = treatment or therapy; UCLA = University of California at Los Angeles; UI = uninsured; USC = usual source of care; USRDS = U.S. Renal Data System; VA = Department of Veterans Affairs.

C

Glossary and Acronyms

GLOSSARY

Adjusted, adjustment   In a statistical analysis, the process of manipulating or stratifying the values of independent variables so as to minimize their confounding influence on the relationship or association between an independent variable of interest and the dependent variable.

Association   A correlation or relationship that may or may not be causal, for example when events occur more frequently together than one would expect by chance alone.★

Bias   "Any systematic error in the design, conduct or analysis of a study that results in a mistaken estimate of an exposure's effect on the risk of disease" (Gordis, 1996, p. 183).

Bivariate analysis   A statistical method to characterize the relationship between an independent variable that measures an exposure or treatment (e.g., a potential cause) and a dependent variable that measures an outcome or effect.

Causality   A relationship that may exist between an exposure or treatment (cause) and an outcome (effect), depending in part on the strength of the association between exposure or treatment and outcome.

★Adapted from the Academy for Health Services Research and Health Care Policy glossary at http://www.academyhealth.org/publications.glossary.pdf, accessed February 4, 2002.

Chronic disease A disease that has one or more of the following characteristics: is permanent; leaves residual disability; is caused by nonreversible physiological damage; requires special training of the patient for rehabilitation; or may be expected to require a long period of supervision, observation, or care.★

Confidence interval (CI) A numeric range estimated with a specific degree of confidence or probability to include a value. Conventionally reported confidence intervals are ranges in which the actual value of the estimated variable can be expected to fall 95 or 99 percent of the time, corresponding to probabilities that a difference or significant result is due to chance of 5 percent and 1 percent, respectively (p ≤.05; p ≤.01). In reporting quantified results throughout this report (e.g., odds ratios or relative risks), if the confidence interval is *not* given, point estimates have *at least* a 95 percent probability of being statistically significant. Confidence intervals are given for findings reported with lesser levels of statistical significance.

Confounder A variable that is associated with an exposure or treatment of interest and, as a result, influences the relationship between the exposure or treatment and an outcome. The ability to adjust or analytically control for the presence of a confounder depends on how well this variable is measured.

Cost sharing Any provision of a health insurance policy that requires the insured individual to pay some portion of medical expenses. The general term includes deductibles, copayments, and coinsurance.★

Covariate A variable that is related to or associated with the study variable(s) of interest.

Cross-sectional Describes a research study in which measurements are collected and comparisons made among populations at one point in time.

Experimental Describes a study design, for example, a randomized clinical trial, where researchers use a defined study population, randomly assign members of the population to exposure or treatment and control groups, control the timing of the exposure or treatment, and influence the timing of measurements.

Hazard ratio, Cox proportional hazard rate A comparative measure of the strength of a relationship or association between an exposure, intervention, or

---

★Adapted from the Academy for Health Services Research and Health Care Policy glossary at http://www.academyhealth.org/publications.glossary.pdf, accessed February 4, 2002.

treatment (e.g., measured in terms of one or more independent variables) and an outcome (e.g., measured in terms of a dependent variable) over time for a defined study population divided into exposure and control groups. For example, to estimate the influence of an exposure on the length of time until death (mortality over time), the use of a Cox proportional hazard rate or hazard ratio allows for multivariate analysis of the incremental or proportional difference that each unit of time would be expected to make in increasing or reducing the risk of mortality. In this example, the mortality hazard ratio, or incidence of mortality estimated at one moment in time, is defined as the relative risk of mortality for persons in an exposure group compared with the relative risk of mortality for members of a control group.

Health-related quality of life (HRQOL) A research construct developed by the Centers for Disease Control and Prevention to help monitor progress in achieving national health objectives. It has been used in the Behavioral Risk Factor Surveillance System surveys since 1993 and, since 2000, in the National Health and Nutrition Examination Survey. Its core element consists of four questions that encompass general self-reported health status, the number of unhealthy days within a recent time period (e.g., the month before the interview) for both physical and mental dimensions, and restricted activity days.

Incidence A measure of the probability of a disease or an outcome's occurrence, defined as the number of new cases within a defined time period for a specific population divided by the total number in the population (Gordis, 1996).

Longitudinal Describes a research study in which measurements are collected and comparisons made among populations over time.

Medically indigent Persons who cannot afford needed health care because of insufficient income and/or lack of adequate health insurance. Indigent care consists of health services provided to the poor or those unable to pay. Since many indigent patients are not eligible for federal or state programs, the costs that are covered by Medicaid are generally recorded separately from indigent care costs.*

Multivariable or multivariate analysis A statistical method to characterize the relationship among at least two independent variables that measure exposures or treatments (e.g., potential causes) and a dependent variable that measures an outcome or effect.

---

*Adapted from the Academy for Health Services Research and Health Care Policy glossary at http: //www.academyhealth.org/publications.glossary.pdf, accessed February 4, 2002.

Observational   Describes a research study with a nonexperimental design, in which researchers gather observations or measurements while not intentionally affecting the conditions of exposure, the treatment of the study population, or the timing of measurements.

Odds ratio (OR)   A comparative measure of the strength of a relationship or association between an exposure or treatment and an outcome for two populations, where the baseline incidence of the outcome in these groups may not be known. In this report, it is the relative odds of either (1) developing the outcome for an uninsured group, compared with the odds for an insured group, or (2) having been uninsured for a group with an outcome, compared with the odds for a control population. For example, if the odds of receiving a Pap test are 2:1 in a group of uninsured women (i.e., two of every three women, or 67 percent, receive the test) and the odds are 4:1 in a group of women with insurance (i.e., four of every five women, or 80 percent, receive the test), the odds ratio of uninsured compared to insured women is 0.5 (2:1/4:1). The OR is not a good estimate of the relative risk (the probability of been screened in the uninsured group divided by the probability of being screened in the insured group) because screening is not a rare event.

Predictor, independent predictor   In a statistical analysis, an independent variable (e.g., that measures an exposure or treatment) that is shown to be likely to influence or predict the value of a dependent variable (e.g., an outcome).

Prevalence   A measure of how common a disease or condition is within a population, defined as the number of cases in the population at a specified time divided by the number of persons in the population at that same time (Gordis, 1996).

Quasi-experimental   Describes a research study, for example, a natural experiment, whose design combines experimental and nonexperimental aspects. Typically, researchers cannot control the timing of the intervention or exposure whose effects are being measured, or the random assignment of a defined group of study subjects, but they can influence the timing of measurements.

Randomized trial   Describes a research study in which the members of a defined group of subjects are randomly assigned to at least two groups for the purpose of analysis: a treatment or intervention group and a control group.

Relative risk (RR)   A comparative measure of the strength of a relationship or association between an exposure, intervention, or treatment and an outcome for a defined study population, where the baseline incidence of the outcome is known. It is expressed as the ratio of two risks, namely, the rate of a disease or condition of interest in the treated portion of the population, divided by the rate in an untreated or control portion of the population. A value of one means that the rates in both portions are the same.★

Selection bias In research studies, a systematic error in analysis that results when study subjects are not assigned randomly among treatment and control groups.

Statistically significant See definition of *Confidence interval.*

ACRONYMS

AMI	acute myocardial infarction
ASOC	Survey of Aging, Status and the Sense of Control
BRFSS	Behavioral Risk Factor Surveillance System
CABG	coronary artery bypass graft
CBE	clinical breast exam
CDC	Centers for Disease Control and Prevention
CI	confidence interval
CPS	Current Population Survey
ED	emergency department
EPO	erythropoietin
ESRD	end-stage renal disease
FFS	fee for service
FOBT	fecal occult blood test
FPL	federal poverty level
HAART	highly active antiretroviral therapy
HCSUS	HIV Cost and Services Utilization Study
HCUP	Healthcare Cost and Utilization Project
HMO	health maintenance organization
HRQOL	health-related quality of life
ICU	intensive care unit
IOM	Institute of Medicine
ISS	injury severity score

★Adapted from the Academy for Health Services Research and Health Care Policy glossary at http://www.academyhealth.org/publications.glossary.pdf, accessed February 4, 2002.

LOS   length of stay

MEPS   Medical Expenditure Panel Survey

NCHS   National Center for Health Statistics
NHANES   National Health and Nutrition Examination Survey
NHIS   National Health Interview Survey
NMES   National Medical Expenditure Survey
NNRTI   nonnucleoside reverse transcriptase inhibitor
NRMI   National Registry of Myocardial Infarction

OR   odds ratio

PI   protease inhibitor
PTCA   percutaneous transluminal coronary angioplasty

RR   relative risk
RWJF   The Robert Wood Johnson Foundation

SCHIP   State Children's Health Insurance Program
SEER   Surveillance, Epidemiology, and End Results Program
SES   socioeconomic status
SMI   severe mental illness

UCSF   University of California at San Francisco
USRDS   United States Renal Data System

VA   Department of Veterans Affairs

D

Estimates of Excess Mortality Among Uninsured Adults

This appendix illustrates, at the level of the U.S. population overall, the magnitude of differences in the mortality experience of insured and uninsured adults based on the mortality results reported in several of the studies reviewed. The Committee presents these population-level extrapolations of the differing risks of premature death for insured and uninsured adults in order to provide a sense of the actual implications of the differential access and care that adults without health insurance experience at the level of society overall. This exercise is performed for the overall adult population and for adults with one of three conditions whose mortality risks have been studied in conjunction with health insurance: hypertension, breast cancer, and HIV infection.

The ranges of estimates within each category and their widely varying population-level magnitudes serve to demonstrate how the impact of health insurance status on overall mortality depends on

- the prevalence and mortality risks of the condition,
- the age and demographic distributions of those afflicted by the condition, and
- the effectiveness of appropriate health care services in reducing mortality from it.

OVERALL MORTALITY RISK

Two longitudinal studies reviewed in Chapter 3, one of 13–17 years' duration and the other of 5 years' follow-up, support the use of an estimate of a higher overall mortality risk for uninsured adults of 25 percent (Franks et al., 1993a;

Sorlie et al., 1994). Table D.1 presents the population parameters on which the estimate of overall excess mortality among uninsured adults are based. The total number of deaths estimated within each age group for 2000 (based on the mortality rates for 1999) is a function of the different mortality rates for the insured and the uninsured populations. By applying the mortality hazard ratio of 1.25 to the uninsured population estimate for each age group, the number of excess deaths among the uninsured population can be calculated. For example, for those ages 25–34, the overall deaths (40,548) = $(0.79)(x) + (0.21)(1.25)(x)$, where 0.79 and 0.21 represent the proportions of the population with and without health insurance, respectively[1]; 1.25 is the mortality hazard ratio of uninsured to insured; and x is the number of deaths expected across the population if everyone had the mortality rate of the insured population. By solving for x, in this case $x = 38,617$, and subtracting that from the actual (estimated) number of deaths (40,548), the excess deaths among uninsured 25–34 year olds is 1,930.

Repeating this calculation for each age group, excess deaths among uninsured adults ages 25–64, based on a 25 percent higher mortality risk, can be estimated to be in the range of 18,000 each year. This calculation makes a number of simplifying assumptions, including that the incremental mortality risk of being uninsured is constant over the 25-64 age range, but it gives an order of magnitude to the potential impact of uninsurance on mortality. For comparison, diabetes accounts for between 15,000 and 16,000 deaths each year and cerebrovascular disease (e.g., stroke) between 18,000 and 19,000 among 25–64 year olds (CDC, 2000b).

Hypertension

More than 23 million U.S. residents between 25 and 65 are estimated to have either diagnosed or undiagnosed hypertension, based on the National Health and Nutrition Examination Survey III (Hyman and Pavlik, 2001). The rate of uninsurance for the general population in this age group is 16 percent (Table D.1). If adults between ages 25 and 65 who have hypertension are as likely to lack health insurance as the overall population in this age range, then about 3.68 million adults with hypertension can be expected to be uninsured.

The RAND Health Insurance Experiment documented a 10 percent lower overall mortality risk for adults with hypertension in insurance plans with no cost sharing compared to those in plans with any cost sharing, due to better hypertension treatment (Newhouse et al., 1993). This 10 percent value is used here as an estimate of the differential overall mortality between uninsured and insured adults ages 25–64 with hypertension.[2] If these 3.68 million uninsured adults with hyper-

---

[1]Actual calculation carried out with more significant digits.

[2]The assumption that the difference in hypertension detection, treatment, and control between the free-care and any-cost-sharing groups in the RAND study is comparable to the difference for adults

TABLE D.1 Estimated excess deaths among uninsured adults 25–64 for 2000

Age	U.S. Population 2000[a] (millions)	Uninsured Population 2000 (millions)	Percent Uninsured (within age group)	Deaths per Million 1999 (estimated)	Total Deaths Estimated for 2000 Population	Uninsured Excess Deaths Estimated for 2000 Population
25–34	37.440	7.926	(21)	1,083	40,548	1,930
35–44	44.780	6.938	(15)	1,992	89,202	3,431
45–54	38.040	4.571	(12)	4,273	162,545	4,734
55–64	23.784	3.248	(14)	10,219	243,049	8,219
Total	144.044	22.683	(16)	3,717	535,344	18,314

[a]Census estimates, Current Population Survey March supplement, Web page, accessed January 09, 2002. Available at http://ferret.bls.census.gov/macro/0332001/health/h01_001.htm.

tension were to experience a 10 percent reduction in their mortality risk as a result of gaining health insurance, calculating from the general population mortality rate for adults ages 25–64 (3,717 per million, as presented in Table D.1), the excess deaths among uninsured adults due to unidentified and undertreated hypertension are about 1,300 or 1,400 each year (10 percent of 3,717 = 372 excess deaths/million population, multiplied by 3.68 million = 1,369).

Breast Cancer

Approximately 40,200 women died of breast cancer in 2001, an estimated 16,560 of them under age 65 (41.2 percent of breast cancer deaths in 1997 occurred in women under age 65) (NCI–SEER, 2001). Using an uninsured rate of 7.55 percent for women diagnosed with breast cancer (the uninsured rate estimated for adults under 65 with all forms of cancer, based on unpublished Medical Expenditure Panel Survey [MEPS] data for 1997),[3] the excess mortality for uninsured women with breast cancer can be calculated. Using the study findings reported in Chapter 3 of a 30 to 50 percent greater risk of dying among uninsured women (Ayanian et al., 1993; Lee-Feldstein et al., 2000; Roetzheim et al., 2000a), the number of excess deaths among uninsured women that are attributable to their higher risk is in the range of 360 to 600 each year. This estimate is conservative because it does not take into account those women who were uninsured at the time the disease developed but who gained coverage (most probably Medicaid) at some point thereafter. If the uninsured rate for all women in the 50–64 year-old age range, 13–14 percent were used in the estimate, the number of excess deaths due to uninsurance would almost double.

HIV Infection

Approximately 20 percent of HIV-infected adults are uninsured, based on HIV Cost and Services Utilization Study interviews in 1996–1997 (Goldman et al., 2001). The 12-month mortality rate for HIV-infected adults over this same time period was 5 percent. In 1998, 12,750 deaths attributable to HIV occurred in adults ages 25–64 (CDC, 2000b). HIV-infected adults who have health insurance have been estimated to have a 71–85 percent lower risk of dying within six months than do those who are uninsured (Goldman et al., 2001). By assuming that

---

with and without health insurance is speculative but reasonable. (The estimated service utilization difference between insured adults who face no cost sharing and those who face cost sharing is likely to be smaller than that between uninsured adults and adults with any form of health insurance. The results of the quasi-experimental Medi-Cal study reported in Chapter 3 also support this assumption (Lurie et al., 1984; 1986).

[3]MEPS data provided to the Institute of Medicine (IOM) by the Center for Cost and Financing Studies, Agency for Healthcare Research and Quality, December 2001.

the one-year differential mortality between insured and uninsured HIV-infected adults is similar to the six-month differential, the number of excess deaths annually among HIV-infected adults without insurance can be estimated by solving the following equation: 12,750 [actual HIV deaths in 1998] = 0.8(0.29 *or* 0.15)(x) + 0.2(x), where (x) is the number of deaths among uninsured adults. After solving for (x), the difference between (x) and the range represented by 0.15(x) to 0.29(x) constitutes the excess mortality among uninsured adults with HIV infection. This amounts to 1,200 to 1,500 excess deaths among the uninsured with HIV each year.

SUMMARY

These estimates of condition-specific excess deaths annually among uninsured adults:

- 1,300–1,400 due to unidentified and undertreated hypertension,
- 360–600 among women with breast cancer, and
- 1,200–1,500 among HIV-infected adults,

are meant to be illustrative. They provide a sense of how the overall mortality risk for uninsured adults, estimated here to be on the order of 18,000 excess deaths among uninsured adults annually, is comprised of elevated mortality rates across many disease categories. All of these excess deaths among uninsured adults occur among relatively young Americans, those under the age of 65.

E

Biographical Sketches

COMMITTEE ON THE CONSEQUENCES OF UNINSURANCE
SUBCOMMITTEE ON THE HEALTH OUTCOMES OF THE UNINSURED

Mary Sue Coleman, Ph.D., *Co-chair,* is president of the University of Iowa and president of the University of Iowa Health Systems. She holds academic appointments as professor of biochemistry in the College of Medicine and professor of biological sciences in the College of Liberal Arts. Dr. Coleman served as provost and vice president for academic affairs at the University of New Mexico (1993–1995) and dean of research, and vice chancellor at the University of North Carolina at Chapel Hill (1990–1992). She was both faculty member and Cancer Center administrator at the University of Kentucky in Lexington for 19 years, where her research focused on the immune system and malignancies. Dr. Coleman is a member of the Institute of Medicine (IOM) and a Fellow of the American Association for the Advancement of Science. She serves on the Iowa Governor's Strategic Planning Council, the Board of Trustees of the Universities Research Association, the Board of Governors of the Warren G. Magnuson Clinical Center at the National Institutes of Health, and other voluntary advisory bodies and corporate boards.

Arthur L. Kellermann, M.D., M.P.H., *Co-chair,* is professor and director, Center for Injury Control, Rollins School of Public Health, Emory University, and professor and chairman, Department of Emergency Medicine, School of

Medicine, Emory University. Dr. Kellerman has served as principal investigator or co-investigator on several research grants, including federally funded studies of handgun-related violence and injury, emergency cardiac care, and the use of emergency room services. Among his many awards and distinctions, he is a fellow of the American College of Emergency Physicians (1992); is the recipient of a meritorious service award from the Tennessee State Legislature (1993); the Hal Jayne Academic Excellence Award from the Society for Academic Emergency Medicine (1997); and was elected to membership in the IOM (1999). In addition, Dr. Kellermann is a member of the Editorial Board of the journal *Annals of Emergency Medicine*, and has served as a reviewer for the *New England Journal of Medicine*, the *Journal of the American Medical Association*, and the *American Journal of Public Health*.

Ronald M. Andersen, Ph.D.,★ is the Fred W. and Pamela K. Wasserman Professor of Health Services and professor of sociology at the University of California, Los Angeles School of Public Health. He teaches courses in health services organization, research methods, evaluation, and leadership. Dr. Andersen received his Ph.D. in sociology at Purdue University. He has studied access to medical care for his entire professional career of 30 years. Dr. Andersen developed the Behavioral Model of Health Services Use that has been used extensively both nationally and internationally as a framework for utilization and cost studies of general populations, as well as special studies of minorities, low income, children, women, the elderly, oral health, the homeless, and the HIV-positive population. He has directed three national surveys of access to care and has led numerous evaluations of local and regional populations and programs designed to promote access to medical care. Dr. Andersen's other research interests include international comparisons of health services systems, graduate medical education curricula, physician health services organization integration, and evaluations of geriatric and primary care delivery. He is a member of the IOM and was on the founding Board of the Association for Health Services Research. He has been chair of the Medical Sociology Section of the American Sociological Association. In 1994 he received the association's Leo G. Reeder Award for Distinguished Service to Medical Sociology; in 1996 he received the Distinguished Investigator Award from the Association for Health Services Research; and in 1999 he received the Baxter Allegiance Health Services Research Prize.

John Z. Ayanian, M.D., M.P.P.,★ is an associate professor of medicine and health care policy at Harvard Medical School and Brigham and Women's Hospital, where he practices general internal medicine. His research focuses on quality of care and access to care for major medical conditions, including colorectal cancer and myocardial infarction. He has extensive experience in the use of cancer

---

★Member of the Subcommittee on the Health Outcomes of the Uninsured

bestowed on her, Dr. Hernández was named by *Modern Healthcare* magazine as one of the top 10 health care leaders for the next century. Dr. Hernández is a graduate of Yale University, Tufts School of Medicine, and the JFK School of Government at Harvard University. She is on the faculty of the University of California, San Francisco (UCSF) School of Medicine and maintains an active clinical practice at San Francisco General Hospital in the AIDS Clinic.

Willard G. Manning, Ph.D., is professor in the Department of Health Studies, Pritzker School of Medicine, and in the Harris School of Public Policy, at the University of Chicago. His primary research focus has been the effects of health insurance and alternative delivery systems on the use of health services and health status. He is an expert in statistical issues in cost-effectiveness analysis and small-area variations. His recent work has included examination of mental health services use and outcomes in a Medicaid population, and cost-effectiveness analysis of screening and treating depression in primary care. Dr. Manning is a member of the IOM.

David O. Meltzer, M.D., Ph.D.,★ is an assistant professor in the Department of Medicine and an associate faculty member of the Harris School and the Department of Economics at the University of Chicago. Dr. Meltzer's research explores problems in health economics and public policy. His recent work has focused on the theoretical foundations of medical cost-effectiveness analysis, including issues such as accounting for future costs due to the extension of life and the empirical validity of quality-of-life assessment, which he has examined in the context of diabetes and prostate cancer. Another major area of study examines the effects of managed care and medical specialization on the cost and quality of care, especially in teaching hospitals. Dr. Meltzer is the recipient of numerous awards: the National Science Foundation Graduate Fellowship in Economics, the Lee Lusted Prize of the Society for Medical Decision Making, the Health Care Research Award of the National Institute for Health Care Management, and the Robert Wood Johnson Generalist Physician Award. He is also a faculty research fellow for the National Bureau of Economic Research and has served on a panel that examined the Future of Medicare for the National Academy of Social Insurance and served on the IOM Organ Procurement and Transplantation Policy Committee.

James J. Mongan, M.D., is president and chief operating officer of Massachusetts General Hospital. He was previously executive director, Truman Medical Center, and dean, University of Missouri-Kansas City School of Medicine. Dr. Mongan served as assistant surgeon general in the Department of Health and

---

★Member of the Subcommittee on the Health Outcomes of the Uninsured.

Human Services (DHHS), as former associate director for health and human resources, Domestic Policy Staff, the White House; and as former deputy assistant secretary for Health Policy, Department of Health, Education and Welfare. Dr. Mongan is chair of the Task Force on the Future of Health Insurance for Working Americans, a nonpartisan effort of the Commonwealth Fund to address the implications of the changing U.S. work force and economy for the availability and affordability of health insurance, and is a member of the Kaiser Family Foundation Board and the Kaiser Commission on the Underserved and the Uninsured.

Cynthia D. Mulrow, M.D., M.Sc.,★ is clinical professor of medicine at the University of Texas Health Science Center at San Antonio, program director of the Robert Wood Johnson Foundation's Generalist Physician Faculty Scholars Program, and Deputy Editor of *Annals of Internal Medicine*. Dr. Mulrow's editorial board memberships and positions have included the editorial board of the *British Medical Journal*, the *American Journal of Medicine*, and the *ACP Journal Club* and the Clinical Advisory and Editorial Board (electronic and print Evidence-Based Therapeutics Compendium). Dr. Mulrow's expertise in clinical methodology, information synthesis, and systematic reviews also has resulted in invitations to serve on many national and international committees and task forces, including the National Advisory Committee of the Robert Wood Johnson Foundation's Generalist Physician Faculty Scholars Program, the U.S. Preventive Services Task Force, and the Veterans Administration's National Research and Methodology Committee.

Christopher Queram, M.A., has been CEO of the Employer Health Care Alliance Cooperative (The Alliance) of Madison, Wisconsin, since 1993. The Alliance is a purchasing cooperative owned by more than 175 member companies that contracts with providers, manages and reports data, performs consumer education, and designs employer and provider quality initiatives. Prior to his current position, Mr. Queram served as vice president for programs at Meriter Hospital, a 475-bed hospital in Madison. Mr. Queram is a member of the Board of the National Business Coalition on Health and served as board chair for the past two years. He was a member of the President's Advisory Commission on Consumer Protection and Quality in the Health Care Industry. Mr. Queram served as a member of the Planning Committee for the National Quality Forum and continues as convenor of the Purchaser Council of the Forum. He is a member of the Wisconsin Board on Health Information and the Board of the Wisconsin Private Employer Health Care Coverage program. He holds a master's degree in health services administration from the University of Wisconsin at Madison and is a fellow in the American College of Healthcare Executives.

Shoshanna Sofaer, Dr.P.H., is the Robert P. Luciano Professor of Health Care

---

★Member of the Subcommittee on the Health Outcomes of the Uninsured.

Policy at the School of Public Affairs, Baruch College, in New York City. She completed her master's and doctoral degrees in public health at the University of California, Berkeley; taught for six years at the University of California, Los Angeles, School of Public Health; and served on the faculty of George Washington University Medical Center, where she was professor and associate dean for research of the School of Public Health and Health Services, and director of the Center for Health Outcomes Improvement Research. Dr. Sofaer's research interests include providing information to individual consumers on the performance of the health care system; assessing the impact of information on both consumers and the system; developing consumer-relevant performance measures; and improving the responsiveness of the Medicare program to the needs of current and future cohorts of older persons and persons with disabilities. In addition, Dr. Sofaer studies the role of community coalitions in pursuing public health and health care system reform objectives and has extensive experience in the evaluation of community health improvement interventions. She has studied the determinants of health insurance status among the near-elderly, including early retirees. Dr. Sofaer served as Co-Chair of the Working Group on Coverage for Low Income and Non-Working Families for the White House Task Force on Health Care Reform in 1993. Currently, she is co-chair of the Task Force on Medicare of the Century Foundation in New York City, a member of the Board of Health Care Services, IOM, and a member of the AHRQ Health Systems Study Section.

Stephen J. Trejo, Ph.D., is associate professor in the Department of Economics at the University of Texas at Austin. His primary research focus has been in the field of labor economics. He has examined the response of labor market participants to incentives created by market opportunities, government policies, and the institutional environment. Specific research topics include the economic effects of overtime pay regulation; immigrant labor market outcomes and welfare recipiency; the impact of labor unions on compensation, employment, and work schedules; the importance of sector-specific skills; and the relative economic status of Mexican Americans.

Reed V. Tuckson, M.D., is senior vice president of consumer health and medical care enhancement at United Health Group. Formerly, he was senior vice president, professional standards at the American Medical Association. Dr. Tuckson was president of Charles R. Drew University, School of Medicine and Science from 1991 to 1997. From 1986 to 1990, he was commissioner of public health for the District of Columbia. Dr. Tuckson serves on a number of health care, academic, and federal boards and committees and is a nationally known lecturer on topics concerning community-based medicine, the moral responsibilities of health professionals, and physician leadership. He currently serves on the IOM Roundtable on Research and Development of Drugs, Biologics, and Medical Devices and is a member of the IOM.

Edward H. Wagner, M.D., M.P.H., F.A.C.P.,★ is a general internist–epidemiologist and director of the W.A. MacColl Institute for Healthcare Innovation at the Center for Health Studies, Group Health Cooperative of Puget Sound. He is also professor of health services at the University of Washington School of Public Health and Community Medicine. Current research interests include development and testing of population-based care models for diabetes, frail elderly, and chronic illnesses; evaluation of the health and cost impacts of chronic disease and cancer interventions; and interventions to prevent disability and reduce depressive symptoms in older adults. Dr. Wagner has written two books and more than 200 journal articles. He serves on the editorial boards of *Health Services Research* and the *Journal of Clinical Epidemiology*, and acts as a consultant to multiple federal agencies and private foundations. He recently completed a stint as senior advisor on managed care initiatives in the Director's Office of the National Institutes of Health. As of June 1998, he directs Improving Chronic Illness Care (ICIC), a national program of the Robert Wood Johnson Foundation. The overall goal of ICIC is to assist health systems improve their care of chronic illness through quality improvement and evaluation, research, and dissemination. Dr. Wagner is also principal investigator of the Cancer Research Network, a National Cancer Institute funded consortium of 10 health maintenance organizations (HMOs) conducting collaborative cancer effectiveness research.

Lawrence Wallack, Dr.P.H., is professor of public health and director, School of Community Health at Portland State University. He is also Professor Emeritus of Public Health, University of California, Berkeley. Dr. Wallack's primary interest is in the role of mass communication, particularly the news media, in shaping public health issues. His current research is on how public health issues are framed in print and broadcast news. He is principal author of *Media Advocacy and Public Health: Power for Prevention and News for a Change: An Advocate's Guide to Working with the Media*. He is also co-editor of *Mass Communications and Public Health: Complexities and Conflicts*. Dr. Wallack has published extensively on topics related to prevention, health promotion, and community interventions. Specific content areas of his research and intervention work have included alcohol, tobacco, violence, handguns, sexually transmitted diseases, cervical and breast cancer, affirmative action, suicide, and childhood lead poisoning. Dr. Wallack is a member of the IOM Committee on Communication for Behavior Change in the 21st Century: Improving the Health of Diverse Populations.

Robin M. Weinick, Ph.D.,★ is director of intramural research in the Center for Primary Care Research at the Agency for Healthcare Research and Quality. Dr. Weinick led AHRQ's efforts to build research agendas addressing the health care needs of low-income Americans and those residing in urban areas, and led an

---

★Member of the Subcommittee on the Health Outcomes of the Uninsured.

interagency effort to develop a data system for monitoring the status of the health care safety net. She was actively involved with the Medical Expenditure Panel Survey project through various phases of the survey process, including questionnaire design, pretesting, interviewer training, data editing, and data release activities. Dr. Weinick has served as chairperson of several analytic groups contributing to different areas of survey content and data preparation, particularly access to care, health status and conditions, and demographics. Her research focuses on the relationship between families and health, as well as on access to care and populations at risk of not having adequate access to and use of health care services, with particular emphasis on racial and ethnic disparities, children, and the impact of managed care gatekeeping.

Institute of Medicine Staff

Wilhelmine Miller, M.S., Ph.D., is a senior program officer in the Division of Health Care Services. She served as staff to the Committee on Immunization Finance Policy and Practices, conducting and directing case studies of health care financing and public health services. Prior to joining IOM, Dr. Miller was an adjunct faculty member in the Departments of Philosophy at Georgetown University and Trinity College, teaching political philosophy, ethics, and public policy. She received her doctorate from Georgetown, with studies and research in bioethics and issues of social justice. In 1994–1995, Dr. Miller was a consultant to the President's Advisory Committee on Human Radiation Experiments. Dr. Miller was a program analyst in the DHHS for 14 years, responsible for policy development and regulatory review in areas including hospital and HMO payment, prescription drug benefits, and child health. Her M.S. from Harvard University is in health policy and management.

Dianne Miller Wolman, M.G.A., joined the Health Care Services Division of the Institute of Medicine in 1999 as a senior program officer. She directed the study that resulted in the IOM report *Medicare Laboratory Payment Policy: Now and in the Future*, released in 2000. Her previous work experience in the health field has been varied and extensive, focused on finance and reimbursement in insurance programs. She came from the General Accounting Office, where she was a senior evaluator on studies of the Health Care Financing Administration, its management capacity, and its oversight of Medicare contractors. Prior to that, she was a reimbursement policy specialist at a national association representing nonprofit providers of long-term care services. Her earlier positions included policy analysis and management in the office of the secretary in the DHHS, and work with a peer review organization, a governor's task force on access to health care, and a third-party administrator for very large health plans. In addition, she was policy director for a state Medicaid rate setting commission. She has a master's degree in government administration from Wharton Graduate School, University of Pennsylvania.

Lynne Page Snyder, Ph.D., M.P.H., is a program officer in the IOM Division of Health Care Services. She came to IOM from DHHS, where she worked as a public historian, documenting and writing about past federal activities in medicine, health care, and public health. In addition, she has worked for the Social Science Research Council's Committee on the Urban Underclass and served as a graduate fellow at the Smithsonian Institution's National Museum of American History. She has published on twentieth century health policy, occupational and environmental health, and minority health. Current research interests include health literacy and access to care by low-income seniors. She earned her doctorate in the history and sociology of science from the University of Pennsylvania (1994), working under Rosemary Stevens, and received her M.P.H. from the Johns Hopkins School of Hygiene and Public Health (2000).

Tracy McKay, B.A., is a research associate in the IOM Division of Health Care Services. She has worked on several projects, including the National Roundtable on Health Care Quality; Children, Health Insurance, and Access to Care; Quality of Health Care in America; and a study on non-heart-beating organ donors. She has assisted in the research for The National Quality Report on Health Care Delivery, Immunization Finance Policies and Practices, and Extending Medicare Coverage for Preventive and Other Services and helped develop this project on the consequences of uninsurance from its inception. Ms. McKay received her B.A. in sociology from Vassar College in 1996.

Ryan Palugod, B.S., is a senior program assistant in the IOM Division of Health Care Services. Prior to joining the project staff in 2001, he worked as an administrative assistant with the American Association of Homes and Services for the Aging. He graduated with honors from Towson University with a degree in health care management in 1999.

Consultant to the Committee on the Consequences of Uninsurance

Jennifer S. Haas, M.D., M.P.H., is assistant professor of medicine and researcher in the Institute for Health Policy Studies, University of California, San Francisco. Dr. Haas is an attending physician in the General Medical Clinic. Her research interests include women's health, evaluation of the quality of medical care, access to medical care, and the health impacts both of health insurance and of socioeconomic status and race and ethnicity. She is affiliated with the Medical Effectiveness Research Center at UCSF and the Institute for Health Policy Studies. She graduated from Harvard Medical School, completed residency training in primary care medicine in the Department of General Internal Medicine at San Francisco General Hospital, and received an M.P.H. from the Harvard School of Public Health.

References

Academy for Health Services Research and Health Policy. 2000. "Glossary of Terms Commonly Used In Health Care." Web page, accessed February 4, 2002. Available at www.academyhealth. org/publications.glossary.

Adler, Nancy E., W. Thomas Boyce, Margaret A. Chesney, S. Cohen, et al. 1994. Socioeconomic Status and Health: The Challenge of the Gradient. *American Psychology* 49(1):15–24.

Agency for Health Care Policy and Research (AHCPR). 1993. *Depression in Primary Care: Treatment of Major Depression.* U.S. Department of Health and Human Services, Rockville, MD.

American College of Physicians–American Society of Internal Medicine. 1999. *No Health Insurance? It's Enough to Make You Sick.* Philadelphia, PA: American College of Physicians–American Society of Internal Medicine.

American Diabetes Association. 2000. Standards of Medical Care for Patients with Diabetes Mellitus. *Diabetes Care* 23(Suppl. 1):S32–S42.

American Heart Association. 2001. *2002 Heart and Stroke Statistical Update.* American Heart Association, Dallas, TX.

Andersen, Ronald, and Pamela Davidson. 2001. Improving Access to Care in America: Individual and Contextual Indictators. In: Ronald Andersen, Thomas Rice, and Gerald Kominski (eds.) *Changing the U.S. Health Care System: Key Issues in Health Services, Policy and Management.* San Francisco, CA: Jossey-Bass. Pp. 3–30.

Andersen, Ronald, Samuel Bozzette, Martin Shapiro, Patricia St. Clair, et al. 2000. Access of Vulnerable Groups to Antiretroviral Therapy Among Persons in Care for HIV Disease in the United States. *Health Services Research* 35(2):389–416.

Apter, Andrea J., Susan T. Reisine, Glenn Affleck, Erik B.A. Barrows, et al. 1999. The Influence of Demographic and Socioeconomic Factors on Health-Related Quality of Life in Asthma. *Journal of Allergy & Clinical Immunology* 103(1, Pt. 1):72–78.

Ayanian, John Z., Betsy A. Kohler, Toshi Abe, and Arnold M. Epstein. 1993. The Relation Between Health Insurance Coverage and Clinical Outcomes Among Women with Breast Cancer. *New England Journal of Medicine* 329(5):326–331.

Ayanian, John Z., Joel S. Weissman, Eric C. Schneider, Jack A. Ginsburg, et al.. 2000. Unmet Health Needs of Uninsured Adults in the United States. *Journal of the American Medical Association* 284(16):2061–2069.

Baker, David W., Martin F. Shapiro, and Claudia L. Schur. 2000. Health Insurance and Access to Care for Symptomatic Conditions. *Archives of Internal Medicine* 160(9):1269–1274.

Baker, David W., Joseph J. Sudano, Jeffrey M. Albert, Elaine A. Borawski, et al. 2001. Lack of Health Insurance and Decline in Overall Health in Late Middle Age. *New England Journal of Medicine* 345(15):1106–1112.

Baker, Richard S., Neil L. Watkins, Roy Wilson, M. Bazargan, et al. 1998. Demographic and Clinical Characteristics of Patients with Diabetes Presenting to an Urban Public Hospital Ophthalmology Clinic. *Ophthalmology* 105(8):1373–1379.

Bazelon Center for Mental Health Law/Milbank Memorial Fund. 2000. *Effective Public Management of Mental Health Care: Views from States*. New York, NY: Milbank Memorial Fund.

Becker, Gary. 2001. Effects of Being Uninsured on Ethnic Minorities' Management of Chronic Illness. *Western Journal of Medicine* 175(1):19–23.

Beckles, Gloria L. A., Michael M. Engelgau, K. M. Venkat Narayan, William H. Herman, et al. 1998. Population-Based Assessment of the Level of Care Among Adults with Diabetes in the U.S. *Diabetes Care* 21(9):1432–1438.

Behera, S. K., Marilyn A. Winkleby, and R. Collins. 2000. Low Awareness of Cardiovascular Disease Risk Among Low-Income African-American Women. *American Journal of Health Promotion* 14(5):301–305, iii.

Bennett, Charles L., Ronnie D. Horner, Robert A. Weinstein, Gordon Dickinson, et al. 1995. Racial Differences in Care Among Hospitalized Patients With *Pneumocystis carinii* Pneumonia in Chicago, New York, Los Angeles, Miami, and Raleigh-Durham. *Archives of Internal Medicine* 155(8):1586–1592.

Berg, John W., Ronald Ross, and Howard B. Latourette. 1977. Economic Status and Survival of Cancer Patients. *Cancer* 39(2):467–477.

Berk, Marc L., and Claudia L. Schur. 1998. Access to Care: How Much Difference Does Medicaid Make? *Health Affairs* 17(3):169–180.

Bindman, Andrew B., Kevid Grumbach, Dennis Osmand, Miriam Komaromy, et al. 1995. Preventable Hospitalizations and Access to Care. *Journal of the American Medical Association* 274(4):305–311.

Bindman, Andrew B., Kevin Grumbach, Dennis Osmond, Karen Vranizan, et al. 1996. Primary Care and Receipt of Preventive Services. *Journal of General Internal Medicine* 11(5):269–276.

Bing, Eric G., Amy M. Kilbourne, Ronald A. Brooks, Ellen F. Lazarus, et al. 1999. Protease Inhibitor Use Among a Community Sample of People With HIV Disease. *Journal of Acquired Immune Deficiency Syndrome* 20(5):474–480.

Blustein, Jan, Raymond R. Arons, and Steven Shea. 1995. Sequential Events Contributing to Variations in Cardiac Revascularization Rates. *Medical Care* 33(8):864–880.

Blustein, Jan, Karla Hanson, and Steven Shea. 1998. Preventable Hospitalizations and Socioeconomic Status. *Health Affairs* 17(2):177–189.

Bonnie, Richard J., Carolyn E. Fulco, and Catheryn T. Liverman (eds.) 1999. *Reducing the Burden of Injury. Advancing Prevention and Treatment*. Washington, DC: National Academy Press.

Bozzette, Samuel A., Sandra H. Berry, Naihua Duan, Martin R. Frankel, et al. 1998. The Care of HIV-Infected Adults in the United States. *New England Journal of Medicine* 339(26):1897–1904.

Bozzette, Samuel A., Geoffrey Joyce, Daniel F. McCaffrey, Arleen A. Leibowitz, et al. 2001. Expenditures for the Care of HIV-Infected Patients in the Era of Highly Active Antiretroviral Therapy. *New England Journal of Medicine* 344(11):817–823.

Braveman, Paula, Mylo Schaaf, Susan Egerter, Trude Bennett, et al. 1994. Insurance-Related Differences in the Risk of Ruptured Appendix. *New England Journal of Medicine* 331(7):444–449.

Breen, Nancy, Diane Wagener, Martin L. Brown, William Davis, et al. 2001. Progress in Cancer Screening Over a Decade. Results of Cancer Screening from the 1987, 1992 and 1998 National Health Interview Surveys. *Journal of the National Cancer Institute* 93(22):1704–1713.

Broaddus, Matthew, and Leighton, Ku. 2000. Nearly 95 Percent of Low-Income Uninsured Children Now Are Eligible for Medicaid or SCHIP. Web page, Accessed May 7, 2001. Available at http://www.cbpp.org.

Broman, Clifford L. 1996. The Health Consequences of Racial Discrimination: A Study of African Americans. *Ethnicity and Disease* 6(1–2):148–153.

Brook, Robert H., John E. Ware, William H. Rogers, Emmett B. Keeler, et al. 1983. Does Free Care Improve Adults' Health? Results from a Randomized Controlled Trial. *New England Journal of Medicine* 309(23):1427–1434.

Brooks, John M., Mark McClellan, and Herbert S. Wong. 2000. The Marginal Benefits of Invasive Treatments for Acute Myocardial Infarction: Does Insurance Coverage Matter? *Inquiry* 37(1):75–90.

Brown, Margaret E., Andrew B. Bindman, and Nicole Lurie. 1998. Monitoring the Consequences of Uninsurance: A Review of the Methodologies. *Medical Care Research and Review* 55(2):177–210.

Burack, Robert C., Phyllis A. Gimotty, William Stengle, L. Warbase, et al. 1993. Patterns of Use of Mammography Among Inner-City Detroit Women: Contrasts Between a Health Department, HMO, and Private Hospital. *Medical Care* 31(4):322–334.

Burstin, Helen R., Stuart R. Lipsitz, and Troyen A. Brennan. 1992. Socioeconomic Status and Risk for Substandard Medical Care. *Journal of the American Medical Association* 268(17):2383–2387.

Burstin, Helen R., Katherine Swartz, Anne C. O'Neill, E. John Orav, et al. 1998. The Effect of Change of Health Insurance on Access to Care. *Inquiry* 35:389–397.

Burt, Vicki L., Paul Whelton, Edward J. Roccella, Clarice Brown, et al. 1995. Prevalence of Hypertension in the U.S. Adult Population: Results from the Third National Health and Nutrition Exam Survey, 1988-1991. *Hypertension* 25(3):303–313.

Bush, Ruth A., and Robert D. Langer. 1998. The Effects of Insurance Coverage and Ethnicity on Mammography Utilization in a Postmenopausal Population. *Western Journal of Medicine* 168(4):236–240.

Canto, John G., William J. Rogers, Yuan Zhang, Jeffrey M. Roseman, et al. 1999. The Association Between the On-Site Availability of Cardiac Procedures and the Utilization of Those Services for Acute Myocardial Infarction by Payer Group. *Clinical Cardiology* 22(8):519–524.

Canto, John G., William J. Rogers, William J. French, Joel M. Gore, et al. 2000. Payer Status and the Utilization of Hospital Resources in Acute Myocardial Infarction. *Archives of Internal Medicine* 160(6):817–823.

Carlisle, David M., Barbara D. Leake, and Martin F. Shapiro. 1997. Racial and Ethnic Disparities in the Use of Cardiovascular Procedures: Associations with Type of Health Insurance. *American Journal of Public Health* 87(2):263–267.

Carlisle, David M., and Barbara D. Leake. 1998. Differences in the Effect of Patients' Socioeconomic Status on the Use of Invasive Cardiovascular Procedures Across Health Insurance Categories. *American Journal of Public Health* 88(7):1089–1092.

Carpenter, Charles C. J., Margaret A. Fischl, Scott M. Hammer, Martin S. Hirsch, et al. 1998. Antiretroviral Therapy for HIV Infection in 1998: Updated Recommendations of the International AIDS Society-USA Panel. *Journal of the American Medical Association* 280(1):78–86.

———. 1996. Antiretroviral Therapy for HIV Infection in 1996. *Journal of the American Medical Association* 276, (2):146–154.

Carrasquillo, Olveen, David U. Himmelstein, Steffie Woolhandler, and David H. Bor. 1998. Can Medicaid Mangaged Care Provide Continuity of Care to New Medicaid Enrollees? An Analysis of Tenure on Medicaid. *American Journal of Public Health* 88(3):464–466.

Carrasquillo, Olveen, Angeles I. Carrasquillo, and Steven Shea. 2000. Health Insurance Coverage of Immigrants Living in the United States. *American Journal of Public Health* 90(6):917–923.

Centers for Disease Control and Prevention (CDC). 1999a. "Chronic Disease Prevention: Chronic Diseases and Conditions, Diabetes." Web page, Accessed March 5, 2001. Available at http://www.cdc.gov/nccdphp/diabetes.htm.

————. 1999b. *Chronic Diseases and Their Risk Factors: The Nation's Leading Causes of Death*. U.S. Department of Health and Human Services, Washington, DC.

————. 2000a. "Chronic Disease Prevention: Heart Disease and Health Promotion." Web page, accessed 26 November 26, 2001. Available at http://www.cdc.gov/od/perfplan/2000 viiheart.htm.

————. 2000b. Deaths: Final Data for 1998. *National Vital Statistics Reports* 48(11):1–106.

————. 2001a. "HIV/AIDS Surveillance Report, 2000". Web page, accessed October 25, 2001. Available at HtmlResAnchor http://www.cdc.gov/hiv.

————. 2001b. Mortality from Coronary Heart Disease and Acute Myocardial Infarction—United States, 1998. *Morbidity and Mortality Weekly Report* 50(6):90–93.

————. 2002. Socioeconomic Status of Women With Diabetes—United States, 2000. *Morbidity and Mortality Weekly Report* 51(7):147–148, 159.

Cetjin, Helen E., Eugene Komaroff, L. Stewart Massad, Abner Korn, et al. 1999. Adherence to Colposcopy Among Women With HIV Infection. *Journal of Acquired Immune Deficiency Syndrome* 22(3):247–252.

Chao, Ann, Michael J. Thun, Eric J. Jacobs, S. Jane Henley, et al. 2000. Cigarette Smoking and Colorectal Cancer Mortality in the Cancer Prevention Study II. *Journal of the National Cancer Institute*. 92(23):1888–1896.

Chin, Marhsall H., Steven B. Auerback, Sandy Cook, James F. Harrison, et al. 2000. Quality of Diabetes Care in Community Health Centers. *American Journal of Public Health* 90(3):431–434.

Clark, Rodney, Norman B. Anderson, Vernessa R. Clark, and David R. Williams. 1999. Racism as a Stressor for African Americans: A Biopsychosocial Model. *American Psychologist* 54(10):805–816.

Coffield, Ashley B., Michael V. Maciosek, J. Michael McGinnis, Jeffrey R. Harris, et al. 2001. Priorities Among Recommended Clinical Preventive Services. *American Journal of Preventive Medicine* 21(1):1–9.

Cohen, S., David A. Tyrrell, and Andrew P. Smith. 1991. Psychological Stress and Susceptibility to the Common Cold. *New England Journal of Medicine* 325(9):606–612.

Collins, Karen Scott, Allyson G. Hall, and Charlotte Neuhaus. 1999. *U.S. Minority Health: A Chartbook*. New York: The Commonwealth Fund.

Cooper-Patrick, Lisa, Rosa M. Crum, Laura A. Pratt, William W. Eaton, et al. 1999. The Psychiatric Profile of Patients with Chronic Disease Who Do Not Receive Regular Medical Care. *International Journal of Psychiatry* 29(2):165–180.

Cummings, Doyle M., Lauren Whetstone, Amy Shende, and David Weismiller. 2000. Predictors of Screenings Mammography: Implications for Office Practice. *Archives of Family Medicine* 9(9):870–875.

Cunningham, Peter J., and Heidi Whitmore. 1998. *How Well Do Communities Perform on Access?* Washington, DC: Center for Studying Health System Change.

Cunningham, Peter J., Jerome M. Grossman, Robert F. St. Peter, and Cara S. Lesser. 1999. Managed Care and Physicians' Provision of Charity Care. *Journal of the American Medical Association* 281(12):1087–1092.

Cunningham, William E., Ron D. Hays, Kevin W. Williams, Keith C. Beck, et al. 1995. Access to Medical Care and Health-Related Quality of Life for Low-Income Persons with Symptomatic Human Immunodeficiency Virus. *Medical Care* 33(7):739–754.

Cunningham, William E., David M. Mosen, Ron D. Hays, Ronald M. Andersen, et al. 1996. Access to Community-Based Medical Services and Number of Hospitalizations Among Patients with HIV Disease: Are They Related? *Journal of Acquired Immune Deficiency Syndrome and Human Retrovirology* 13(4):327–335.

Cunningham, William E., Ronald M. Andersen, Mitchell H. Katz, Michael D. Stein, et al. 1999. The Impact of Competing Subsistence Needs and Barriers on Access to Medical Care for Persons with Human Immunodeficiency Virus Receiving Care in the United States. *Medical Care* 37(12):1270–1281.

Cunningham, William E., Leona E. Markson, Ronald M. Andersen, Stephen Crystal, et al. 2000. Prevalence and Predictors of Highly Active Antiretroviral Therapy Use in Patients with Infection in the United States. *Journal of Acquired Immune Deficiency Syndrome* 25(2):115–123.

Curtis, J. Randall, Wylie Burke, Adam W. Kassner, and Moira L. Aitken. 1997. Absence of Health Insurance Is Associated With Decreased Life Expectancy in Patients With Cystic Fibrosis. *American Journal of Respiratory Critical Care Medicine* 155(6):1921–1924.

Cutler, David, Mark McClellan, and Joseph Newhouse. 1998. The Costs and Benefits of Intensive Treatment for Cardiovascular Disease. *NBER Working Paper Series*. National Bureau of Economic Research, Cambridge, MA.

Cutler, David M., E.L. Glaeser, and J.L. Vigdor. 1999. The Rise and Decline of the American Ghetto. *Journal of Political Economy*: 455.

Daumit, Gail, Judith A. Hermann, Josef Coresh, and Neil R. Powe. 1999. Use of Cardiovascular Procedures Among Black Persons and White Persons: A 7-Year Nationwide Study in Patients with Renal Disease. *Annals of Internal Medicine* 130(3):173–182.

Daumit, Gail L., Judith A. Hermann, and Neil R. Powe. 2000. Relation of Gender and Health Insurance to Cardiovascular Procedure Use in Persons with Progression of Chronic Renal Disease. *Medical Care* 38(4):354–365.

Davidoff, Amy, Bowen Garrett, and Alshadye Yemane. 2001. Medicaid-Eligible Adults Who Are Not Enrolled: Who Are They and Do They Get the Care They Need? *New Federalism: Issues and Options for States*. Series A, No. A-48. The Urban Institute, Washington, DC.

Davis, Ronald M., Edward G. Wagner, and Trish Groves. 2000. Advances in Managing Chronic Disease: Research, Performance, and Quality Improvement Are Key. *British Medical Journal* 320(7234):525–526.

DeCorte, P., Jeannette Gunther, T. Harrison-Woodside., David Jewell, et al. 1995. Health Insurance: Impact on Hospitalization Rates for Asthma. *Nursingconnections* 8(3):33–42.

Depression Guideline Panel. 1993. *Depression in Primary Care: Treatment of Major Depression*. Rockville, MD: U.S. Department of Health and Human Services, Agency for Health Care Policy and Research.

Dixon, Lori Beth, Marilyn A. Winkleby, and K. L. Radimer. 2001. Dietary Intakes and Serum Nutrients Differ Between Adults From Food-Insufficient Families: Third National Health and Nutrition Examination Survey, 1988–1994. *Journal of Nutrition* 131(4):1232–1246.

Doescher, Mark P., Peter Franks, Jessica S. Banthin, and Carolyn M. Clancy. 2000. Supplemental Insurance and Mortality in Elderly Americans. *Archives of Family Medicine* 9:251–257.

Doyle, Joseph J. 2001. *Does Health Insurance Affect Treatment Decisions & Patient Outcomes? Using Automobile Accidents as Unexpected Health Shocks*. Chicago: University of Chicago, unpublished MS.

Druss, Benjamin G., and Robert A. Rosenheck. 1998. Mental Disorders and Access to Medical Care in the United States. *American Journal of Psychiatry* 155(12):1775–1777.

Druss, Benjamin G., W. David Bradford, Robert A. Rosenheck, Martha J. Radford, et al. 2001. Quality of Medical Care and Excess Mortality in Older Patients With Mental Disorders. *Archives of General Psychiatry* 58(6):565–572.

Eger, Renee R., and Jeffrey F. Peipert. 1996. Risk Factors for Noncompliance in a Colposcopy Clinic. *The Journal of Reproductive Medicine* 41(9):671–674.

Eisenberg, John M. and Elaine J. Power. 2000. Transforming Insurance Coverage Into Quality Health Care. *JAMA* 284(16):2100–2107.

Ell, Kathleen, Julian Haywood, Eugene Sobel, Maria deGuzman, et al. 1994. Acute Chest Pain in African Americans: Factors in the Delay in Seeking Emergency Care. *American Journal of Public Health* 84(6):965–970.

Elo, Irma T. and Samuel H. Preston. 1996. Educational Differentials in Mortality: United States, 1979–1985. *Social Science and Medicine* 42(1):47–57.

Evans, Jennifer L., Philip C. Nasca, Mark S. Baptiste, P.P. Lillquist, et al. 1998. Factors Associated With Repeat Mammography in a New York State Public Health Screening Program. *Journal of Public Health and Management Practice* 4(5):63–71.

Fairbrother, Gerry, Heidi Park, and M. Gusmano. 2002. How Community Health Centers Are Coping With Their Uninsured Caseloads. *National Association of Community Health Centers 27th Policy and Issues Forum*. Washington, DC.

Faulkner, Lisa A. and Helen Halpin Schauffler. 1997. The Effect of Health Insurance Coverage on the Appropriate Use of Recommended Clinical Preventive Services. *American Journal of Preventive Medicine* 13(6):453–458.

Ferrante, Jeanne M., Eduardo Gonzalez, Richard G. Roetzheim, Naazneen Pal, et al. 2000. Clinical and Demographic Predictors of Late-Stage Cervical Cancer. *Archives of Family Medicine* 9(5):439–445.

Ferrer, Robert L. 2001. A Piece of My Mind: Within the System of No-System. *Journal of the American Medical Association* 286(20):2513–2514.

Fishman, Eliot. 2001. Aging Out of Coverage: Young Adults With Special Health Needs. *Health Affairs* 20(6):254-267.

Fish-Parcham, Cheryl. 2001. *Getting Less Care: The Uninsured with Chronic Health Conditions*. Washington, DC: Families USA Foundation.

Fleishman, John A., and Vincent Mor. 1993. Insurance Status Among People with AIDS: Relationships with Sociodemographic Characteristics and Service Use. *Inquiry* 30(2):180–188.

Ford, Earl S., Robert K. Merritt, Gregory W. Heath, Kenneth E. Powell, et al. 1991. Physical Activity Behaviors in Lower and Higher Socioeconomic Status Populations. *American Journal of Epidemiology* 133(12):1246–1256.

Ford, Earl S., Julie C. Will, Martine A. De Proost, and Ali H.Mokdad. 1998. Health Insurance Status and Cardiovascular Disease Risk Factors Among 50-64-Year-Old U.S. Women: Findings from the Third National Health and Nutrition Examination Survey. *Journal of Women's Health* 7(8):997–1006.

Franks, Peter, Carolyn M. Clancy, and Marthe R. Gold. 1993a. Health Insurance and Mortality. Evidence from a National Cohort. *Journal of the American Medical Association* 270(6):737–741.

Franks, Peter, Carolyn M. Clancy, Marthe R. Gold, Paul A. Nutting, et al. 1993b. Health Insurance and Subjective Health Status: Data from the 1987 National Medical Expenditure Survey. *American Journal of Public Health* 83(9):1295–1299.

Freeman, Howard E., and Christopher R. Corey. 1993. Insurance Status and Access to Health Services Among Poor Persons. *Health Services Research* 28(5):531–541.

Fronstin, Paul. 2000. *Sources of Health Insurance and Characteristics of the Uninsured: Analysis of the March 2000 Current Population Survey*. Employee Benefit Research Institute, Washington, DC.

Fronstin, Paul. 2001a. *Employment-Based Health Benefits: Trends and Outlook*. Employee Benefit Research Institute, Washington, DC.

Fronstin, Paul. 2001b. *Sources of Health Insurance and Characteristics of the Uninsured: Analysis of the March 2001 Current Population Survey*, Employee Benefit Research Institute, Washington, DC.

Fronstin, Paul, and Virginia Reno. 2001. *Recent Trends in Retiree Health Benefits and the Role of COBRA Coverage*, National Academy of Social Insurance, Washington, DC.

Fuentes-Afflick, Elena, Nancy A. Hessol, and Eliseo J. Perez-Stable. 1999. Testing the Epidemiologic Paradox of Low Birth Weight in Latinos. *Archives of Pediatrics & Adolescent Medicine* 153(2):147–153.

Gabel, Jon. 1999. Job-Based Health Insurance, 1977–1998: The Accidental System Under Scrutiny. *Health Affairs* 18(6):62–74.

Garrett, Bowen, and John Holahan. 2000. Health Insurance Coverage After Welfare. *Health Affairs* 19(1):175–184.

Gaskin, Darrell J., and Catherine Hoffman. 2000. Racial and Ethnic Differences in Preventable Hospitalizations Across 10 States. *Medical Care Research and Review* 57(Suppl. 1):85–107.

Goldman, Dana P., Jayanta Bhattcharya, Daniel F. McCaffrey, Naihua Duan, et al. 2001. Effect of Insurance on Mortality in an HIV-Positive Population in Care. *Journal of the American Statistical Association* 96(455): 883–894.

Gordis, Leon. 1996. *Epidemiology*. Philadelphia: W.B. Saunders and Co.

Gordon, Nancy P., Thomas G. Rundall, and Laurence Parker. 1998. Type of Health Care Coverage and the Likelihood of Being Screened for Cancer. *Medical Care* 36(5):636–645.

Gorey, Kevin M., Eric Holowaty, Gordon Fehringer, Ethan Laukkanen, et al. 1997. An International Comparison of Cancer Survival: Metropolitan Toronto, Ontario and Honolulu, Hawaii. *American Journal of Public Health* 90(12):1866–1872.

Greenberg, E. Robert, Christopher G. Chute, Therese A. Stukel, John A. Baron, et al. 1988. Social and Economic Factors in the Choice of Lung Cancer Treatment. *New England Journal of Medicine* 318(10):612–617.

Gu, Ken, Catherine C. Cowie, and Maureen I. Harris. 1998. Mortality in Adults With and Without Diabetes in a National Cohort of the U.S. Population, 1971–1993. *Diabetes Care* 21(7):1138–1145.

Guralnik, Jack M., Kenneth C. Land, Dan Blazer, and Gerda G. Fillenbaum. 1993. Educational Status and Active Life Expectancy Among Older Blacks and Whites. *New England Journal of Medicine* 329(2):110–116.

Haan, Mary, Gary A. Kaplan, and Teresa Camacho. 1987. Poverty and Health. Prospective Evidence from the Alameda County Study. *American Journal of Epidemiology* 125(6):989–998.

Haas, Jennifer S., and Lee Goldman. 1994. Acutely Injured Patients with Trauma in Massachusetts: Differences in Care and Mortality by Insurance Status. *American Journal of Public Health* 84(10):1605–1608.

Haas, Jennifer S., Paul D. Cleary, Edward Guadagnoli, Christopher Fanta, et al. 1994. The Impact of Socioeconomic Status on the Intensity of Ambulatory Treatment and Health Outcomes After Hospital Discharge for Adults with Asthma. *Journal of General Internal Medicine* 9(3):121–126.

Haas, Jennifer S., and Nancy E. Adler. 2001. The Causes of Vulnerability: Disentangling the Effects of Race, Socioeconomic Status and Insurance Coverage on Health. Background paper prepared for the Committee on the Consequences of Uninsurance.

Hadley, Jack, Earl P. Steinberg, and Judith Feder. 1991. Comparison of Uninsured and Privately Insured Hospital Patients. *Journal of the American Medical Association* 265(3):374–379.

Haffner, Steven M. 2000. Coronary Artery Disease in Patients with Diabetes. *New England Journal of Medicine* 342(14):1040–1042.

Hafner-Eaton, Chris. 1993. Physician Utilization Disparities Between the Uninsured and Insured. Comparisons of the Chronically Ill, Acutely Ill, and Well Nonelderly Populations. *Journal of the American Medical Association* 269(6):787–792.

Hahn, Beth, and Ann Barry Flood. 1995. No Insurance, Public Insurance, and Private Insurance: Do These Options Contribute to Differences in General Health? *Journal of Health Care for the Poor and Underserved* 6(1):41–59.

Haley, Jennifer M., and Stephen Zuckerman. 2000. *Health Insurance, Access, and Use: United States. Tabulations from the 1997 National Survey of America's Families*. The Urban Institute, Washington, DC.

Hamilton, Barton, Vivian Ho, and H. Paarsch. 1997. The Distribution of Outpatient Services in Canada and the U.S.: An Empirical Model of Physician Visits. Olin School of Business, St. Louis, MO.

Harris, Maureen I. 1999. Racial and Ethnic Differences in Health Insurance Coverage for Adults with Diabetes. *Diabetes Care* 22(10):1679–1682.

Hayward, Rodney A., Martin F. Shapiro, Howard E. Freeman, and Christopher R. Corey. 1988. Who Gets Screened for Cervical and Breast Cancer? *Archives of Internal Medicine* 148(5):1177–1181.

Ho, Vivian, Barton H. Hamilton, and Leslie L. Roos. 2000. Multiple Approaches to Assessing the Effects of Delays for Hip Fracture Patients in the United States and Canada. *Health Services Research* 34(7):1499–1518.

Hoffman, Catherine, and Mary Pohl. 2000. *Health Insurance Coverage in America. 1999 Data Update.* Washington, DC: Kaiser Commission on Medicaid and the Uninsured.

Hoffman, Catherine, Cathy Schoen, Diane Rowland, and Karen Davis. 2001. Gaps in Health Coverage Among Working-Age Americans and the Consequences. *Journal of Health Care for the Poor and Underserved* 12(3):273–289

Holahan, John, and Brenda Spillman. 2002. Health Care Access for Uninsured Adults: A Strong Safety Net is Not the Same as Insurance. *New Federalism: National Survey of America's Families*, Series B, No. B-42. The Urban Institute, Washington, DC.

Holcombe, Randall F., and Jason Griffin. 1993. Effect of Insurance Status on Pain Medication Prescriptions in a Hematology/Oncology Practice. *Southern Medical Journal* 86(2):151–156.

Hsia, Judith, Elizabeth Kemper, Catarina Kiefe, Jane Zapka, et al. 2000. The Importance of Health Insurance as a Determinant of Cancer Screening: Evidence from the Women's Health Initiative. *Preventive Medicine* 31:261–270.

Huttin, Christine, John F. Moeller, and Randall S. Stafford. 2000. Patterns and Costs for Hypertension Treatment in the United States. *Clinical Drug Investigation* 20(3):181–195.

Hyman, David J., and Valory N. Pavlik. 2001. Characteristics of Patients with Uncontrolled Hypertension in the United States. *The New England Journal of Medicine* 345(7):479–486.

Idler, Ellen L., Stanislav V. Kasl, and Jon H. Lemke. 1990. Self-Evaluated Health and Mortality Among the Elderly in New Haven, Connecticut, and Iowa and Washington Counties. *American Journal of Epidemiology* 131(1):91–103.

Institute of Medicine (IOM). 2000a. *America's Health Care Safety Net. Intact but Endangered.* Washington, DC: National Academy Press.

———. 2000b. *Promoting Health: Intervention Strategies from Social and Behavioral Research.* Brian D. Smedley, and S. Leonard Syme (eds.). Washington, DC: National Academy Press.

———. 2001a. *Coverage Matters: Insurance and Health Care.* Washington, DC: National Academies Press.

———. 2001b. *Crossing the Quality Chasm; A Health System for the 21st Century.* Washington, DC: National Academy Press.

———. 2002. *Unequal Treatment: Confronting Racial and Ethnic Disparities in Health Care.* Brian D. Smedley, Adrienne Y. Stith, and Alan R. Nelson (eds.). Washington, DC: National Academy Press.

Jennings-Dozier, Kathleen, and Deirdre Lawrence. 2000. Sociodemographic Predictors of Adherence to Annual Cervical Cancer Screening in Minority Women. *Cancer Nursing* 23(5):350–356.

Jeste, Dilip V., and Jurgen Unuetzer. 2001. Improving the Delivery of Care to the Seriously Mentally Ill. *Medical Care* 39(9):907–909.

Joint National Committee on Prevention, Detection Evaluation and Treatment of High Blood Pressure. 1997. The Sixth Report of the Joint National Committee on Prevention, Detection, Evaluation, and Treatment of High Blood Pressure. *Archives of Internal Medicine* 157(21):2413–2446.

Joyce, Geoffrey F., Dana P. Goldman, Arleen Leibowitz, David Carlisle, et al. 1999. Variation in Inpatient Resource Use in the Treatment of HIV: Do the Privately Insured Receive Better Care? *Medical Care* 37(3):220–227.

The Kaiser Commission on Medicaid and the Uninsured. 2000. *In Their Own Words: The Uninsured Talk About Living Without Health Insurance*, The Kaiser Commission on Medicaid and the Uninsured, Washington, DC.

Kaiser Family Foundation–Health Research and Educational Trust (HRET). 2000. *Employer Health Benefits, 2000. Annual Survey.* Washington, DC.

Karlson, Elizabeth W., Lawrence H. Daltroy, Robert A. Lew, Elizabeth A. Wright, et al. 1995. The Independence and Stability of Socioeconomic Predictors of Morbidity in Systemic Lupus Erythematosus. *Arthritis & Rheumatism* 38(2):267-273.

Kasper, Judith D., Terence A. Giovannini, and Catherine Hoffman. 2000. Gaining and Losing Health Insurance: Strengthening the Evidence for Effects of Access to Care and Health Outcomes. *Medical Care Research and Review* 57(3):298-318.

Katz, Mitchell H., Andrew B. Bindman, Dennis Keane, and Allen K. Chan. 1992. CD4 Lymphocyte Count as an Indicator of Delay in Seeking Human Immunodeficiency Virus-Related Treatment. *Archives of Internal Medicine* 152:1501-1504.

Katz, Mitchell H., Sophia W. Chang, Susan P. Buchbinder, Nancy A. Hessol, et al. 1995. Health Insurance and Use of Medical Services by Men Infected with HIV. *Journal of Acquired Immune Deficiency Syndrome and Human Retrovirology* 8(1):59-63.

Kausz, Annamaria T., Gregorio T. Obrador, Pradeep Arora, Robin Ruthazer, et al. 2000. Late Initiation of Dialysis Among Women and Ethnic Minorities in the United States. *Journal of the American Society of Nephrology* 11(12):2351-2357.

Keeler, Emmett B., Robert H. Brook, George A. Goldberg, Caren J. Kamberg, et al. 1985. How Free Care Reduced Hypertension in the Health Insurance Experiment. *Journal of the American Medical Association* 254(14):1926-1931.

Kerr, Eve A., and Albert L. Siu. 1993. Follow-Up After Hospital Discharge: Does Insurance Make a Difference? *Journal of Health Care for the Poor and Underserved* 4(3):133-142.

Kessler, Ronald C., Katherine A. McGonagle, Shanyang Zhao, Christopher B. Nelson, et al. 1994. Lifetime and 12-Month Prevalence of DSM-III-R Psychiatric Disorders in the United States: Results from the National Comorbidity Survey. *Archives of General Psychiatry* 51(1):8-19.

Kiecolt-Glaser, Janice K., Gayle G. Page, Phillip T. Marucha, Robert C. MacCallum, et al. 1998. Psychological Influences on Surgical Recovery: Perspectives from Psychoneuroimmunology. *American Psychologist* 53(11):1209-1218.

Kilker, Kristen. 2000. Hypertension: A Common Condition for Older Americans. Washington, DC: National Academy on an Aging Society.

Kington, Raynard S., and James P. Smith. 1997. Socioeconomic Status and Racial and Ethnic Differences in Functional Status Associated with Chronic Diseases. *American Journal of Public Health* 87(5):805-810.

Kinsella, Kevin, and Victoria A. Velkoff. 2001. *An Aging World: 2001*, U.S. Census Bureau, Series P95/01-1. Washington, DC: U.S. Government Printing Office.

Kirkman-Liff, Bradford, and Jennie Jacobs Kronenfeld. 1992. Access to Cancer Screening Services for Women. *American Journal of Public Health* 82(5):733-735.

Kollef, Marin H. 1996. Private Attending Physician Status and the Withdrawal of Life-Sustaining Interventions in a Medical Intensive Care Unit Population. *Critical Care Medicine* 24(6):968-975.

Kollef, Marin H., and Suzanne Ward. 1999. The Influence of Access to a Private Attending Physician on the Withdrawal of Life-Sustaining Therapies in the Intensive Care Unit. *Critical Care Medicine* 27(10):2125-2132.

Komaromy, Miriam, Kevin Grumbach, Michael Drake, et al. 1996. The Role of Black and Hispanic Physicians in Providing Health Care for Underserved Populations. *New England Journal of Medicine* 334(20):1305-1310.

Kozak, Lola Jean, Margaret J. Hall, and Maria F. Owings. 2001. Trends in Avoidable Hospitalizations, 1980-1998. *Health Affairs* 20(2):225-232.

KPMG. 1998. *Health Benefits in 1998.* Arlington, VA: KPMG Peat Marwick.

Kreindel, Sylvia, Ronald Rosetti, Robert Goldberg, Judith Savageau, et al. 1997. Health Insurance Coverage and Outcome Following Acute Myocardial Infarction: A Community-Wide Perspective. *Archives of Internal Medicine* 157(7):758-762.

Krieger, Nancy. 1999. Embodying Inequality: A Review of Concepts, Measures, and Methods for Studying Health Consequences of Discrimination. *International Journal of Health Services* 29(2):295-352.

Krieger, Nancy, Diane L. Rowley, Allen A. Herman, Brian Avery, et al. 1993. Racism, Sexism, and Social Class: Implications for Studies of Health, Disease, and Well-Being. *American Journal of Preventive Medicine* 9(6 Suppl.):82–122.

Krieger, Nancy, J. T. Chen, and Joseph V. Selby. 2001. Class Inequalities in Women's Health: Combined Impact of Childhood and Adult Social Class—A Study of 630 U.S. Women. *Public Health* 115(3):175–185.

Krop, Julie S., Josef Coresh, Lloyd E. Chambless, Eyal Shahar, et al. 1999. A Community-Based Study of Explanatory Factors for the Excess Risk for Early Renal Function Decline in Blacks vs Whites with Diabetes. *Archives of Internal Medicine* 159(15):1777–1783.

Kunst, Anton E., and Johan P. Mackenbach. 1994. The Size of Mortality Differences Associated With Educationl Level in Nine Industrialized Countries. *American Journal of Public Health* 84(6):932–937.

Kuykendall, David H., Michael L. Johnson, and Jane M. Geraci. 1995. Expected Source of Payment and Use of Hospital Services for Coronary Atherosclerosis. *Medical Care* 33(7):715–728.

Leape, Lucian L., Lee H. Hilborne, Robert Bell, Caren Kamberg, et al. 1999. Underuse of Cardiac Procedures: Do Women, Ethnic Minorities, and the Uninsured Fail to Received Needed Revascularization? *Annals of Internal Medicine* 130(3):183–192.

Lee-Feldstein, Anna, Paul J. Feldstein, Thomas Buchmuller, and Gale Katterhagen. 2000. The Relationship of HMOs, Health Insurance, and Delivery Systems to Breast Cancer Outcomes. *Medical Care* 38(7):705–718.

Lehman, Anthony F. 1999. Quality of Care in Mental Health: The Case of Schizophrenia. *Health Affairs* 18(5):52–65.

Lurie, Nicole, N. B. Ward, Martin F. Shapiro, and Robert H. Brook. 1984. Termination from Medi-Cal: Does It Affect Health? *New England Journal of Medicine* 311(7):480–484.

Lurie, Nicole, N. B. Ward, Martin F. Shapiro, Carmen F. Gallego, et al. 1986. Termination of Medi-Cal Benefits: A Followup Study One Year Later. *New England Journal of Medicine* 314(19):1266–1268.

Lynch, John W., George A. Kaplan, Richard D. Cohen, Jussi Kauhanen, et al. 1994. Childhood and Adult Socioeconomic Status as Predictors of Mortality in Finland. *Lancet* 343(8896):524–527.

Lynch, John W., George A. Kaplan, and Sarah J. Shema. 1997. Cumulative Impact of Sustained Economic Hardship on Physical, Cognitive, Psychological, and Social Functioning. *New England Journal of Medicine* 337(26):1889–1895.

MacKenzie, Ellen J., Michael J. Bosse, James F. Kellam, Andrew R. Burgess, et al. 2000. Characterization of Patients With High-Energy Lower Extremity Trauma. *Journal of Orthopaedic Trauma* 14(7):455–466.

Mancini, Mary C., E. M. Penny, M.S. Cush, Kenneth Sweatman, et al. 2001. Coronary Artery Bypass Surgery: Are Outcomes Influenced by Demographics or Ability to Pay? *Annals of Surgery* 233(5):617–622.

Mandelblatt, Jeanne S., Karen Gold, Ann S. O'Malley, Kathryn Taylor, et al. 1999. Breast and Cervix Cancer Screening Among Multiethnic Women: Role of Age, Health, and Source of Care. *Preventive Medicine* 28:418–425.

Marmot, Michael G., George D. Smith, Stephen A. Stansfeld, Chandra Patel, et al. 1991. Health Inequalities Among British Civil Servants: The Whitehall II Study. *Lancet* 337(8754):1387–1393.

Marquis, M. Susan, and Stephen H. Long. 1995. The Uninsured Access Gap: Narrowing the Estimates. *Inquiry* 31(4):405–414.

Massey, D. S., and Nancy A. Denton. 1989. Hypersegregation in U.S. Metropolitan Areas: Black and Hispanic Segregation Along Five Dimensions. *Demography* 26(3):373–391.

Maynard, Charles, Lloyd D. Fisher, Eugene R. Passamani, and T. Pullum. 1986. Blacks in the Coronary Artery Surgery Study (CASS): Race and Clinical Decision Making. *American Journal of Public Health* 76(12):1446–1448.

McAlpine, Donna D., and David Mechanic. 2000. Utilization of Specialty Mental Health Care Among Persons with Severe Mental Illness: The Roles of Demographics, Need, Insurance, and Risk. *Health Services Research* 35(1):277–282.

McBride, Timothy D. 1997. Uninsured Spells of the Poor. Prevalence and Duration. *Health Care Financing Review* 19(1):145–160.

McCaig, Linda F., and Catherine W. Burt. 2001. National Hospital Ambulatory Medical Care Survey: 1999 Emergency Department Summary. *Advance Data from Vital and Health Statistics*, No. 320. Hyattsville, MD: National Center for Health Statistics.

Meyer, Madonna Harrington, and Eliza K. Pavalko. 1996. Family, Work, and Access to Health Insurance Among Mature Women. *Journal of Health and Social Behavior* 37(4):311–325.

Millman, Michael (ed.) 1993. *Access to Health Care in America.* Washington, DC: National Academy Press.

Mills, Robert J. 2000. Health Insurance Coverage: 1999. *Current Population Reports.* Washington, DC: U.S. Census Bureau.

————. 2001. Health Insurance Coverage: 2000. *Current Population Reports.* Washington, DC: U.S. Census Bureau.

Monheit, Alan C., and Jessica Primoff Vistnes. 2000. Race/Ethnicity and Health Insurance Status: 1987 and 1996. *Medical Care Research and Review* 57(Suppl. 1):11–35.

Monheit, Alan C., Jessica Primoff Vistnes, and John M. Eisenberg. 2001. Moving to Medicare: Trends in the Health Insurance Status of Near-Elderly Workers, 1987–1996. *Health Affairs* 20(2):204–213.

Mor, Vincent, John Fleishman, Marguerite Dresser, and John Piette. 1992. Variations in Health Service Use Among HIV-Infected Patients. *Medical Care* 30(1):17–29.

Moran, William P., Stuart J. Cohen, John S. Preisser, James L. Wofford, et al. 2000. Factors Influencing Use of the Prostate-Specific Antigen Screening Test in Primary Care. *American Journal of Managed Care* 6(3):315–324.

Mort, Elizabeth A., Jennifer N. Edwards, David W. Emmons, Karen Convery, et al. 1996. Physician Response to Patient Insurance Status in Ambulatory Care Clinical Decision-Making. *Medical Care* 34(8):783–797.

Mosen, David M., Neil S. Wenger, Martin F. Shapiro, Ronald M. Andersen, et al. 1998. Is Access to Medical Care Associated with Receipt of HIV Testing and Counseling? *AIDS Care* 10(5):617–628.

Mossey, Jana M., and Ellen Shapiro. 1982. Self-Rated Health: A Predictor of Mortality Among the Elderly. *American Journal of Public Health* 72(8):800–808.

Murray, Christopher J. L., and Alan D. Lopez (eds). 1996. *The Global Burden of Disease: A Comprehensive Assessment of Mortality and Disability from Diseases, Injuries, and Risk Factors in 1990 and Projected.* Cambridge, MA: Harvard University Press.

Mutchler, Jan E., and Jeffrey A. Burr. 1991. Racial Differences in Health and Health Care Service Utilization in Later Life: The Effect of Socioeconomic Status. *Journal of Health and Social Behavior* 32(4):342–356.

Narrow, William E., Darrel A. Regier, Grayson Norquist, Donald S. Rae, et al. 2000. Mental Health Service Use by Americans with Severe Mental Illnesses. *Social Psychiatry and Psychiatric Epidemiology* 35(4):147–155.

Narrow, William E., Donald S. Rae, Lee N. Robins, and Darrel A. Regier. 2002. Revised Prevalence Estimates of Mental Disorders in the United States. *Archives of General Psychiatry* 59(2):115–123.

Nathens, Avery B., Ronald V. Maier, Michael K. Copass, and Gregory J. Jurkovich. 2001. Payer Status: The Unspoken Triage Criterion. *Journal of Trauma* 50(5):776–783.

National Academy on an Aging Society (NAAS). 1999. Challenges for the 21st Century: Chronic and Disabling Conditions. *Chronic Conditions: A Challenge for the 21st Century.* Washington, DC.

National Cancer Institute–Surveillance, Epidemiology and End Results Program (NCI–SEER). 2001. *SEER Cancer Statistics Review, 1973–1998*, National Cancer Institute, Bethesda, MD, http://seer.cancer.gov/Publications/CSR1973_1998/.

National Center for Health Statistics (NCHS). 2001. *Urban and Rural Health Chartbook: Health, United States, 2001*. National Center for Health Statistics, Hyattsville, MD.

National Cholesterol Education Program (NCEP). 1993. Summary of the Second Report of the National Cholesterol Education Program (NCEP) Expert Panel on Detection, Evaluation, and Treatment of High Blood Cholesterol in Adults (Adult Treatment Panel II). *Journal of the American Medical Association* 269(23):3015–3023.

National Kidney Foundation (NKF). 2001. "Kidney Disease Outcomes Quality Initiative Clinical Practice Guidelines." Web page, accessed April 29, 2002. Available at http://www.kidney.org/professionals/doqi/guidelines/doqi_upex.html.

Nauenberg, Eric, and Kisalaya Basu. 1999. Effect of Insurance Coverage on the Relationship Between Asthma Hospitalizations and Exposure to Air Pollution. *Public Health Reports* 114(2):135–148.

Nelson, David E., Betsy Thompson, Shayne D. Bland, and Richard Rubinson. 1999. Trends in Perceived Cost as a Barrier to Medical Care, 1991–1996. *American Journal of Public Health* 89(9):1410–1412.

Newacheck, Paul W., Michelle Pearl, Dana C. Hughes, and Neal Halfon. 1998a. The Role of Medicaid in Ensuring Children's Access to Care. *Journal of the American Medical Association* 280(20):1789–1793.

Newacheck, Paul W., Jeffery J. Stoddard, and Dana C. Hughes. 1998b. Health Insurance and Access to Primary Care for Children. *New England Journal of Medicine* 338(8):513–518.

Newhouse, Joseph P., and The Insurance Experiment Group. 1993. *Free for All? Lessons from the RAND Health Insurance Experiment*. Cambridge, MA: Harvard University Press.

Niemcryk, Steve J., Ani Bedros, Katherine M. Marconi, and Joseph F. O'Neill. 1998. Consistency in Maintaing Contact with HIV-Related Service Providers: An Analysis of the AIDS Cost and Services Utilization Study (ACSUS). *Journal of Community Health* 23(2):137–152.

Obrador, Gregorio T., Robin Ruthazer, Arora Pradeep, Annamaria T. Kausz, et al. 1999. Prevalence of and Factors Associated with Suboptimal Care Before Initiation of Dialysis in the United States. *Journal of the American Society of Nephrology* 10(8):1793–1800.

O'Connor, Patrick J., Jay Desai, William A. Rush, Linda Cherney, et al. 1998. Is Having a Regular Provider of Diabetes Care Related to Intensity of Care and Glycemic Control? *Journal of Family Practice* 47(4):290–297.

O'Malley, Ann S., Jeanne Mandelblatt, Karen Gold, Kathleen A. Cagney, et al. 1997. Continuity of Care and the Use of Breast and Cervical Cancer Screening Services in a Multiethnic Community. *Archives of Internal Medicine* 157(13):1462–1470.

O'Malley, Michael S., Jo Anne L. Earp, Sarah T. Hawley, Michael J. Schell, et al. 2001. The Association of Race/Ethnicity, Socioeconomic Status, and Physician Recommendation for Mammography: Who Gets the Message About Breast Cancer Screening? *American Journal of Public Health* 9(1):49–54.

Office of Technology Assessment (OTA). 1992. *Does Health Insurance Make a Difference? Background Paper*. Pub. No. OTA-BP-H-99. Washington, DC: U.S Government Printing Office.

Olfson, Mark, Steven C. Marcus, Benjamin Druss, Lynn Elinson, et al. 2002. National Trends in the Outpatient Treatment of Depression. *Journal of the American Medical Association* 287(2):203–209.

Ostrove, Joan M., Nancy E. Adler, Miriam Kuppermann, and Eugene E. Washington. 2000. Objective and Subjective Assessments of Socioeconomic Status and Their Relationship to Self-Rated Health in an Ethnically Diverse Sample of Pregnant Women. *Health Psychology* 19(6):613–618.

Otten, M. W., Jr., Steven M. Teutsch, David F. Williamson, and James S. Marks. 1990. The Effect of Known Risk Factors on the Excess Mortality of Black Adults in the United States. *Journal of the American Medical Association* 263(6):845–850.

Palacio, Herminia, Caroline H. Shiboski, Edward H. Yelin, Nancy A. Hessol, et al. 1999. Access to and Utilization of Primary Care Services Among HIV-Infected Women. *Journal of Acquired Immune Deficiency Syndromes* 21(4):293–300.

Palta, Mari, Tamara LeCaire, Kathleen Daniels, Guanghong Shen, et al. 1997. Risk Factors for Hospitalization in a Cohort with Type 1 Diabetes. *American Journal of Epidemiology* 146(8):627–636.

Pamuk, Elsie, Diane Makuc, Katherine E. Heck, Cynthia Reuben, et al. 1998. *Socioeconomic Status and Health Chartbook. Health, United States, 1998*, National Center for Health Statistics, Hyattsville, MD.

Pappas, Gregory, Susan Queen, Wilbur Hadden, and Gail Fisher. 1993. The Increasing Disparity in Mortality Between Socioeconomic Groups in the United States, 1960 and 1986. *New England Journal of Medicine* 329(2):103–109.

Pappas, Gregory, Wilbur C. Hadden, Lola Jean Kozak, Gail F. Fisher. 1997. Potentially Avoidable Hospitalizations: Inequities in Rates Between US Socioeconomic Groups. *American Journal of Public Health* 87(5):811–816.

Penson, David F., Marcia L. Stoddard, David J. Pasta, Deborah P. Lubeck, et al. 2001. The Association Between Socioeconomic Status, Health Insurance Coverage, and Quality of Life in Men With Prostate Cancer. *Journal of Clinical Epidemiology* 54(4):350–358.

Perez, Norvin, and Harry H. Tsou. 1995. Prostate Cancer Screening Practices: Differences Between Clinic and Private Patients. *Mount Sinai Journal of Medicine* 62(4):316–321.

Perkins, Carin, William E. Wright, Mark Allen, Steven J. Samuels, et al. 2001. Breast Cancer Stage at Diagnosis in Relation to Duration of Medicaid Enrollment. *Medical Care* 39(11):1224–1233.

Philis-Tsimikas, Athena, and Chris Walker. 2001. Improved Care for Diabetes in Underserved Populations. *Journal of Ambulatory Care Management* 24(1):39–43.

Piette, John D. 2000. Perceived Access Problems Among Patients with Diabetes in Two Public Systems of Care. *Journal of General Internal Medicine* 15(11):797–804.

Pincus, Theodore, Leigh F. Callahan, and R.V. Burkhauser. 1987. Most Chronic Diseases Are Reported More Frequently by Individuals with Fewer Than 12 Years of Formal Education in the Age 18-64 United States Population. *Journal of Chronic Disease* 40(9):865–874.

Pollack, Harold, and Karl Kronebusch. 2001. Health Insurance and Vulnerable Populations. Prepared for University of Michigan conference, Research Initiative on Health Insurance, July 8–10.

Pollitz, Karen. 2001. Extending Health Insurance Coverage for Older Workers and Early Retirees. Pp. 233–254 in *Ensuring Health and Income Security for an Aging Workforce*. Peter P. Budetti, Richard V. Burkhauser, Janice M. Gregory, and H. Allan Hunt (eds.). Kalamazoo, MI: W.E. Upjohn Institute for Employment Research.

Potosky, Arnold L., Nancy Breen, Barry I. Graubard, and P. Ellen Parsons. 1998. The Association Between Health Care Coverage and the Use of Cancer Screening Tests. *Medical Care* 36(3):257–270.

Powe, Neil R., Bernard Jaar, Susan L. Furth, Judith Hermann, et al. 1999. Septicemia in Dialysis Patients: Incidence, Risk Factors, and Prognosis. *Kidney International* 55(3):1081–1090.

Powell-Griner, Eve, Julie Bolen, and Shayne Bland. 1999. Health Care Coverage and Use of Preventive Services Among the Near Elderly in the United States. *American Journal of Public Health* 89(6):882–886.

Preston, Samuel H., and Irma T. Elo. 1995. Are Education Differentials in Adult Mortality Increasing in the United States? *Journal of Aging and Health* 7(4):476–496.

Rabinowitz, Jonathan, Evelyn Bromet, Janet Lavelle, Kimberly Severance, et al. 1998. Relationship Between Type of Insurance and Care During Early Course of Psychosis. *American Journal of Psychiatry* 155(10):1392–1397.

Rabinowitz, Jonathan, Evelyn J. Bromet, Janet Lavelle, Kimberly J. Hornak, et al. 2001. Changes in Insurance Coverage and Extent of Care During the Two Years After First Hospitalization for a Psychotic Disorder. *Psychiatric Services* 52(1):87–91.

Regier, Darrel A., William E. Narrow, Donald S. Rae, Ronald W. Manderscheid, et al. 1993. The De Facto US Mental and Addictive Diorders Service System: Epidemiologic Catchment Area Prospective 1-Year Prevalence Rates of Disorders and Services. *Archives of General Psychiatry* 50(2):85–94.

Reisch, Lisa M., Mary B. Barton, Suzanne W. Fletcher, William Kreuter, et al. 2000. Breast Cancer Screening Use by African Americans and Whites in an HMO. *Journal of General Internal Medicine* 15(4):229–234.

Rhee, Peter M., David Grossman, Frederick Rivara, Charles Mock, et al. 1997. The Effect of Payer Status on Utilization of Hospital Resources in Trauma Care. *Archives of Surgery* 132(4):399–404.

Roetzheim, Richard G., Naazneen Pal, Colleen Tennant, Lydia Voti, et al. 1999. Effects of Health Insurance and Race on Early Detection of Cancer. *Journal of the National Cancer Institute* 91(16):1409–1415.

Roetzheim, Richard G., Eduardo C. Gonzalez, Jeanne M. Ferrante, Naazneen Pal, et al. 2000a. Effects of Health Insurance and Race on Breast Carcinoma Treatments and Outcomes. *Cancer* 89(11):2202–2213.

Roetzheim, Richard G., Naazneen Pal, Eduardo C. Gonzalez, Jeanne M. Ferrante, et al. 2000b. Effects of Health Insurance and Race on Colorectal Cancer Treatments and Outcomes. *American Journal of Public Health* 90(11):1746–1754.

Ross, Catherine E., and John Mirowsky. 2000. Does Medical Insurance Contribute to Socioeconomic Differentials in Health? *Milbank Quarterly* 78(2):291–321.

Ruberman, William, E. Weinblatt, James D. Goldberg, and B.S. Chaudhary. 1991. Psychosocial Influences on Mortality After Myocardial Infarction. *New England Journal of Medicine* 325(9):552–559.

Rucker, Donald W., Troyen A. Brennan, and Helen R. Burstin. 2001. Delay in Seeking Emergency Care. *Academic Emergency Medicine* 8(2):163–169.

Ruggiero, Laurie, Russell E. Glasgow, Janet M. Dryfoos, Joseph S. Rossi, et al. 1997. Diabetes Self-Management. *Diabetes Care* 20(4):568–576.

Sada, Mark J., William J. French, David M. Carlisle, Nisha C. Chandra, et al. 1998. Influence of Payor on Use of Invasive Cardiac Procedures and Patient Outcome After Myocardial Infarction in the United States. *Journal of the American College of Cardiology* 31(7):1474–1480.

Saha, Somnath, Miriam Komaromy, Thomas Koepsell, and Andrew B. Bindman. 1999. Patient-Physician Racial Concordance and the Perceived Quality and Use of Health Care. *Archives of Internal Medicine* 159(9):997–1004.

Samet, Jonathan M., Francesca Dominici, Frank C. Curriero, Ivan Coursac, et al. 2000. Fine Particular Air Pollution and Mortality in 20 U.S. Cities, 1987–1994. *New England Journal of Medicine* 343(24):1742–1749.

Schoen, Cathy, and Catherine DesRoches. 2000. Uninsured and Unstably Insured: The Importance of Continuous Insurance Coverage. *Health Services Research* 35(1):187–206.

Schiff, Robert L., David Ansell, David Goldberg, Stuart Dick, et al. 1998. Access to Primary Care for Patients With Diabetes at an Urban Public Hospital Walk-In Clinic. *Journal of Health Care for the Poor and Underserved* 9(2):170–183.

Schnitzler, Mark A., Dennis L. Lambert, Linda M. Mundy, and Robert S. Woodward. 1998. Variations in Healthcare Measures by Insurance Status for Patients Receiving Ventilator Support. *Clinical Performance of Quality Health Care* 6(1):17–22.

Schulberg, Herbert C., Wayne Katon, Gregory E. Simon, and A. John Rush. 1998. Treating Major Depression in Primary Care Practice: An Update of the Agency for Health Care Policy and Research Practice Guidelines. *Archives of General Psychiatry* 55(12):1121–1127.

Schulman, Kevin A., Jesse A. Berlin, William Harless, Jon F. Kerner, et al. 1999. The Effect of Race and Sex on Physicians' Recommendations for Cardiac Catheterization. *New England Journal of Medicine* 340(8):618–626.

Selden, Thomas M., Jessica S. Banthin, and Joel W. Cohen. 1999. Waiting in the Wings: Eligibility and Enrollment in the State Children's Health Insurance Program. *Health Affairs* 18(2):126–133.

Shapiro, Martin F., Sally C. Morton, Daniel F. McCaffrey, J. Walton Senterfitt, et al. 1999. Variations in the Care of HIV-Infected Adults in the United States. *Journal of the American Medical Association* 281(24):2305–2315.

Shea, Steven, Dawn Misra, Martin Ehrlich, Lesley S. Field, et al. 1992a. Correlates of Nonadherence to Hypertension Treatment in an Inner-City Minority Population. *American Journal of Public Health* 82(12):1607–1612.

Shea, Steven, Dawn Misra, Martin H. Ehrlich, Lesley S. Field, et al. 1992b. Predisposing Factors for Severe, Uncontrolled Hypertension in an Inner-City Minority Population. *New England Journal of Medicine* 327(11):776–781.

Shi, Leiyu. 2000. Type of Health Insurance and Quality of Primary Care Experience. *American Journal of Public Health* 90(12):1848–1855.

Shi, Leiyu. 2001. The Convergence of Vulnerable Characteristics and Health Insurance in the US. *Social Science and Medicine* 53(4):519–529.

Short, Pamela Farley, and Tamra J. Lair. 1994–1995. Health Insurance and Health Status: Implications for Financing Health Care Reform. *Inquiry* 31:425–437.

Short, Pamela Farley, and Vicki A. Freedman. 1998. Single Women and the Dynamics of Medicaid. *Health Services Research* 33(5):1309–1336.

Solis, Julia M., Gary Marks, Melinda Garcia, and David Shelton. 1990. Acculturation, Access to Care, and Use of Preventive Services by Hispanics: Findings from HHANES 1982–1984. *American Journal of Public Health* 80(Suppl.):11–19.

Sorlie, Paul D., Norman J. Johnson, Eric Backlund, and Douglas D. Bradham. 1994. Mortality in the Uninsured Compared with That in Persons with Public and Private Health Insurance. *Archives of Internal Medicine* 154(21):2409–2416.

Sorvillo, Frank, Peter Kerndt, Sylvia Odem, M. Castillon, et al. 1999. Use of Protease Inhibitors Among Persons with AIDS in Los Angeles County. *AIDS Care* 11(2):147–155.

Starfield, Barbara. 1992. Effects of Poverty on Health Status. *Bulletin of the New York Academy of Medicine* 68(1):17–24.

———. 1995. Access—Perceived or Real, and to What? *Journal of the American Medical Association* 274(4):346–347.

———. 1998. Primary Care Visits and Health Policy. *Canadian Medical Association Journal* 159(7):795–796.

Sturm, Roland, and Kenneth B. Wells. 1995. How Can Care for Depression Become More Cost-Effective? *Journal of the American Medical Association* 273(1):51–58.

———. 2000. Health Insurance May Be Improving— But Not for Individuals with Mental Illness. *Health Services Research* 35(1Pt. II):253–262.

Svenson, James E., and Carl W. Spurlock. 2001. Insurance Status and Admission to Hospital for Head Injuries: Are We Part of a Two-Tiered Medical System? *American Journal of Emergency Medicine* 19(1):19–24.

Swartz, Katherine, and Betsey Stevenson. 2001. Health Insurance Coverage of People in the Ten Years Before Medicare Eligibility. Pp. 13–40 in *Ensuring Health and Income Security for an Aging Workforce.* Peter P. Budetti, Richard V. Burkhauser, Janice M. Gergory, and H. Allan Hunt (eds.). Kalamazoo, MI: W.E. Upjohn Institute for Employment Research.

Tin, Jan, and Charita Castro. 2001. Dynamics of Economic Well-Being: Program Participation, 1993 to 1995. Who Gets Assistance? *Current Population Reports.* Washington, DC: U.S. Census Bureau.

Turner, Barbara J., William E. Cunningham, Naihua Duan, Ronald M. Andersen, et al. 2000. Delayed Medical Care After Diagnosis in a US National Probability Sample of Persons Infected With Human Immunodeficiency Virus. *Archives of Internal Medicine* 160(17):2614–2622.

U.S. Department of Health and Human Services (USDHHS). 1998. *Self Reported Use of Mammgraphy and Insurance Status Among Women Aged >40 Years-1991-1992 and 1996-1997.* Morbidity and Mortality Weekly Reports.

———. 1999. "The 1999 HHS Poverty Guidelines." Web page, accessed 24 January 2001. Available at http://aspe.hhs.gov/poverty/99poverty.htm.

———. 2000. *Tracking Healthy People 2010.* Washington, DC: U.S. Government Printing Office.

———. 2001a. *Health, United States, 2001, With Urban and Rural Health Chartbook.* Hyattsville, MD: National Center for Health Statistics, Centers for Disease Control and Prevention.

———. 2001b. *Mental Health: Culture, Race, and Ethnicity-A Supplement to Mental Health: A Report of the Surgeon General.* Rockville, MD: U.S. Department of Health and Human Services, Substance Abuse and Mental Health Services Administration, Center for Mental Health Services.

U.S. Department of Veterans Affairs. 1993. *Clinical Guidelines for Major Depressive Disorder.* Washington, DC: Veterans Health Administration.

U.S. General Accounting Office (GAO). 1998. *Private Health Insurance. Declining Employer Coverage May Affect Access for 55- to 64-Year-Olds.* GAO/HEHE-98-133. Washington, DC.

———. 2001a. *Employer-Sponsored Benefits May Be Vulnerable to Further Erosion.* GAO-01-374. Washington, DC.

———. 2001b. *Gaps in Coverage and Availability.* GAO-02-178T. Washington, DC.

U.S. Preventive Services Task Force. 1996. *Appendix A Task Force Ratings. Guide to Clinical Preventative Services.* Washington, DC.

U.S. Renal Data System (USRDS). 2001. *USRDS 2001 Annual Data Report: Atlas of End-Stage Renal Disease in the United States.* National Institutes of Health, National Institute of Diabetes and Digestive and Kidney Diseases, Bethesda, MD.

U.S. Surgeon General. 1999. *Mental Health: A Report of the Surgeon General.* U.S. Department of Health and Human Services, Substance Abuse and Mental Health Services Administration, Center for Mental Health Services, National Institutes of Health, National Institutes of Mental Health, Rockville, MD.

van Rossum, Caroline T. M., Martin J. Shipley, Hendrike van de Mheen, Diederick E. Grobbee, et al. 2000. Employment Grade Differences in Cause Specific Mortality. A 25 Year Follow Up of Civil Servants From the First Whitehall Study. *Journal of Epidemiology and Community Health* 54(3):178–184.

Vega, William A., and H. Amaro. 1994. Latino Outlook: Good Health, Uncertain Prognosis. *Annual Review of Public Health* 15:39–67.

Wagner, Edward H., Brian T. Austin, and Michael Von Korff. 1996. Organizing Care for Patients with Chronic Illness. *Milbank Quarterly* 74(4):511–543.

Wagner, Todd H., and Sylvia Guendelman. 2000. Healthcare Utilization Among Hispanics: Findings from the 1994 Minority Health Survey. *American Journal of Managed Care* 6(3):355–364.

Waidmann, Timothy A., and Shruti Rajan. 2000. Race and Ethnic Disparities in Health Care Access and Utilization: An Examination of State Variation. *Medical Care Research and Review* 57(Suppl. 1):55–84.

Wang, Philip S., Patricia Berglund, and Ronald C. Kessler. 2000. Recent Care of Common Mental Disorders in the United States. *Journal of General Internal Medicine* 15:284–292.

Wang, Thomas J., and Randall S. Stafford. 1998. National Patterns and Predictors of beta-Blocker Use in Patients With Coronary Artery Disease. *Archives of Internal Medicine* 158(17):1901–1906.

Warner, Margaret, Patricia M. Barnes, and Lois A. Fingerhut. 2000. *Injury and Poisoning Episodes and Conditions; National Health Interview Survey, 1997.* Hyattsville, MD: National Center for Health Statistics.

Weiner, Saul. 2001. 'I Can't Afford That!' Dilemmas in the Care of the Uninsured and Underinsured. *Journal of General Internal Medicine* 16(6):412–418.

Weinick, Robin M., Samuel H. Zuvekas, and Susan K. Drilea. 1997. Access to Health Care—Sources and Barriers: 1996. *MEPS Research Findings No. 3.* AHCPR Pub. No. 98-0001. Rockville, MD: Agency for Health Care Policy and Research. Previously presented at the International Conference on Health Policy Research, Crystal City, VA, December 5–7.

Weinick, Robin M., Samuel H. Zuvekas, and Joel W. Cohen. 2000. Racial and Ethnic Differences in Access to and Use of Health Care Services, 1977 to 1996. *Medical Care Research and Review* 57(Suppl. 1):36–54.

Weissman, Joel and Arnold M. Epstein. 1989. Case Mix and Resource Utilization by Uninsured Hospital Patients in the Boston Metropolitan Area. *Journal of the American Medical Association* 261(24): 3572–3576.

Weissman, Joel S., and Arnold M. Epstein. 1994. *Falling Through the Safety Net: Insurance Status and Access to Health Care*. Baltimore, MD: Johns Hopkins University Press.

Weissman, Joel S., Constantine Gatsonis, and Arnold M. Epstein. 1992. Rates of Avoidable Hospitalization by Insurance Status in Massachusetts and Maryland. *Journal of the American Medical Association* 268(17):2388–2394.

Weissman, Joel S., Robert Stern, Stephen L. Fielding, and Arnold M. Epstein. 1991. Delayed Access to Health Care: Risk Factors, Reasons, and Consequences. *Annals of Internal Medicine* 114(4):325–331.

Weissman, Joel S., Robert S. Stern, and Arnold M. Epstein. 1994. The Impact of Patient Socioeconomic Status and Other Social Factors on Readmission: A Prospective Study in Four Massachusetts Hospitals. *Inquiry* 31(2):163–172.

Whittle, Jeff, Joseph Conigliaro, Chester B. Good, and Monica Joswiak. 1997. Do Patient Preferences Contribute to Racial Differences in Cardiovascular Procedure Use? *Journal of General Internal Medicine* 12(5):267–273.

Williams, David R., and Harold Neighbors. 2001. Racism, Discrimination and Hypertension: Evidence and Needed Research. *Ethnicity and Disease* 11(4):800–816.

Winawer, Sidney J., Robert H. Fletcher, L. Miller, Fiona Godlee, et al. 1997. Colorectal Cancer Screening: Clinical Guidelines and Rationale. *Gastroenterology* 112(2):594–642.

Winkleby, Marilyn A., Darius E. Jatulis, Edmund Frank, and Stephen P. Fortmann. 1992. Socioeconomic Status and Health: How Education, Income, and Occupation Contribute to Risk Factors for Cardiovascular Disease. *American Journal of Public Health* 82(6):816–820.

Woolhandler, Steffie, and David U. Himmelstein. 1988. Reverse Targeting of Preventive Care Due to Lack of Health Insurance. *Journal of the American Medical Association* 259(19):2872–2874.

Yelin, Edward H., Jane S. Kramer, and Wallace V. Epstein. 1983. Is Health Care Use Equivalent Across Social Groups? A Diagnosis-Based Study. *American Journal of Public Health* 73(5):563–571.

Yergan, John, Ann Barry Flood, Paula Diehr, and James P. LoGerfo. 1988. Relationship Between Patient Source of Payment and the Intensity of Hospital Services. *Medical Care* 26(11):1111–1114.

Young, Alexander, Ruth Klap, Cathy Sherbourne, and Kenneth B. Wells. 2001. The Quality of Care for Depressive and Anxiety Disorders in the United States. *Archives of General Psychiatry* 58(1):55–61.

Young, Gary J., and Bruce B. Cohen. 1991. Inequities in Hospital Care, the Massachusetts Experience. *Inquiry* 28: 255–262.

Zambrana, Ruth E., Nancy Breen, Sarah A. Fox, and Mary Lou Gutierrez-Mohamed. 1999. Use of Cancer Screening Services by Hispanic Women: Analyses by Subgroup. *Preventive Medicine* 29:466–477.

Zuvekas, Samuel H., and Robin M. Weinick. 1999. Changes in Access to Care, 1977-1996: The Role of Health Insurance. *Health Services Research* 34(1):271–279.

Zweifel, P. J., and Willard G. Manning. 2000. Consumer Incentives in Health Care. *Handbook of Health Economics*. Anthony J. Culyer and Joseph P. Newhouse (eds.). Amsterdam: Elsevier.